Natural Childcare

*The Macrobiotic Approach to
Raising a Healthy Family*

An *East West Journal* Anthology

EAST WEST BOOKS

BOSTON

EAST WEST HEALTH BOOKS
P.O. Box 1200, 17 Station Street
Brookline, Massachusetts 02147

ISBN 0-936184-01-9

Published in the United States of America

9876543

Designed by LM Sandhaus Madnick
Cover Photo © 1984 Jerry Howard/Positive Images

Distributed by:
East West Health Books, 17 Station Street, Brookline, MA 02147 and
The Talman Co., 150 Fifth Avenue, New York, NY 10011

Table of Contents

Introduction

T his book has been produced in response to popular demand for information on the subjects of macrobiotic pregnancy, birthing, and child care. As an anthology of articles that have appeared in *East West Journal* over the years, it covers many aspects and opinions.

The contributors are mainly parents who have had the courage to bear and raise their children in a way that is different from the dictates of modern medical science. Many families have begun to take responsibility for their own health and education, reducing their dependence on professionals and experts. In this time of rapid degeneration of physical and mental health and social organization, the future of the world itself is at stake, and the care we give our children is a primary investment in ensuring that future. We need to raise a generation of children sound in body and mind, well-integrated and whole, who know how to look after themselves, and also have a deep concern for and sense of belonging to the rest of humanity. A movement has already begun to turn the tide from an impersonal and mechanistic treatment of children to a way based on patterns of natural development and traditional wisdom. We hope this change in orientation will bring about far-reaching and positive effects on society as a whole.

The willingness of these writers to share their experiences, and often their mistakes, provides a wonderful inspiration and guide for other parents and teachers who are looking for a way to re-humanize our child-rearing practices. As macrobiotic families develop their knowledge and understanding through their own experience, we look forward to the continuing use of *East West Journal* as a forum for the exchange of information and ideas.

—Katriona Forrester

Foreword

Few topics have been as exhaustively covered by the publishing industry over the past decade as that of child birth and rearing. There are thousands of titles in print. Dr. Benjamin Spock's classic *Baby and Child Care* continues to sell a quarter of a million copies per year and is now the second best selling book in U.S. history, after The Bible. Books such as pediatrician Dr. T. Berry Brazelton's *Infants and Mothers*, psychologist Dr. Penelope Leach's *The Child Care Encyclopedia*, Frank Caplan's *First Twelve Months of Life*, and others have explored in depth virtually every facet of parenting, from conception to education.

Why then another book on childcare? *Natural Childcare—An East West Journal Anthology* does not intend to be authoritative or encyclopedic in scope, but it does bring a fresh, sometimes controversial viewpoint to a field dominated by "professionals"—M.D.'s, nurses, child psychologists, and the like. It is a book for parents and by parents. It discusses topics such as how to use safe and natural methods of birth control, what to eat for a healthy pregnancy, whether to consider operations such as vasectomy or circumcision, why to breastfeed, what to do when your children want to eat junk foods, and others that are of primary concern to all parents. The traditional macrobiotic approach to these issues is characterized by both a respect for the wisdom of time-tested customs and an openness to the discoveries of modern medical and psychological research.

An open but skeptical approach to the claims of modern medicine is advisable because, until very recently, it threatened to eradicate much of the mystery and drama of raising a family. Birthing was transferred from the home to the hospital and increasingly was characterized by medical intervention. Infant formula replaced mother's milk as the child's first food. Common childhood diseases were subject to increased attempts at management in the form of drugs, repeated office visits, and vaccinations and immunizations. The collected wisdom of grandparents, midwives, and other parents became a neglected resource. The traditional customs associated with having and raising children in other cultures, from the Far East to Latin America, were considered irrelevant.

It is my hope that the following material will help to reverse these trends by bringing to parents a new perspective on the joyful, arduous, and rewarding undertaking of raising children. *Natural Childcare* encourages parents to trust their own intuition and to approach childrearing with a sense not only of responsibility but adventure. Though it contains considerable down-to-earth practical information, more importantly this book seeks to inspire the kind of caring attitude that leads to physical and spiritual growth for the child and parent. On behalf of the many contributors, the writers, editors, and production staff here at *East West Journal*, who worked to bring this anthology together, I hope it serves its purpose as a guidebook for the dynamic process of creating a healthy and happy family. We also encourage the response of parents and other readers of this book, so that we can create an active dialogue in the creation of a new method of parenting, with its roots in traditional wisdom, but its practicality in the present.

—Mark Mayell
Editor, *East West Journal*

Acknowledgements

This book is a collection of articles that have appeared over the past seven years in the *East West Journal*. They were chosen according to their timeliness and value for mothers, fathers, children, and teachers. Katriona Forrester, whose dedication and encouragement were invaluable in making this book a reality, made the initial selection for this collection.

This book would have never been possible without the help of innumerable friends and supporters. I would like to especially thank the primary typists of the manuscript, Mary Colson and Pamela Fuller, whose dedication to learning a computer system allowed us to typeset directly out of the computer. Meg Seaker and Linda Roszak gave invaluable suggestions to make this more of a book and less an anthology. Bob Felt of Redwing Books taught us the simplest way to transfer a complex design to a simple computer-generated typeset manuscript. Without his help this book might still be waiting to be published.

Michio and Aveline Kushi were our primary inspiration and guides in discovering the many natural and commonsense approaches to child care and child rearing. And, of course, the original authors of these articles are also due appreciation for their pioneering spirit and their enthusiasm in sharing their own experiences and discoveries with so many others.

I especially want to thank my family—my wife Barbara, and children Jesse, Daria, Joshua, Molly, and Sean. Without them I wouldn't know anything about child rearing or health, and without their patience and understanding, the many manuscripts that became chapters in this book would never have been written.

I hope that the experiences and suggestions shared by the authors and parents in this book provide as much help for you as it has for us in producing the book.

—Leonard Jacobs
Publisher, *East West Journal*

This book is dedicated to all the children
of the world, who, we hope, will be
happier and healthier as they discover the
traditional wisdom of their ancestors.

Voices of Experience

Women's Health and Pregnancy
The Dynamic Approach of Christiane Northrup, Mother and M.D.

BY TOM MONTE AND LEONARD JACOBS

Christiane Northrup, M.D., is currently working in Portland, Maine, in a six-person private practice center specializing in obstetrics and gynecology. A graduate of Dartmouth Medical School in 1975, she did her residency training at Tufts New England Medical Center, St. Margaret's Hospital, and Cambridge Hospital in the Boston metropolitan area.

In this interview with former *East West Journal* associate editor Tom Monte and publisher Leonard Jacobs Dr. Northrup talks about her experiences working with women and newborn babies, and her growing interest in macrobiotics.

EWJ: *How did you come to macrobiotics?*
Northrup: One day in early 1980, my cousin and I had dinner at the Seventh Inn restaurant in Boston, and she told me that she had become macrobiotic in order to treat her uterine fibroid cysts. I thought, well, that's interesting, I don't know anything about macrobiotics. So I started to ask her the same old questions every M.D. asks: Where do you get your B vitamins? Where do you get protein? Just the usual gross misunderstandings. But if you talk to a dietician, someone trained in nutrition, and you show them the macrobiotic diet, they see no conflict with good nutrition.

Anyway, my cousin sent me some information about macrobiotics and then told me that the East West Foundation and the Kushi Institute were looking for physicians who were interested and perhaps I could meet macrobiotic educator Michio Kushi. I thought I'd like that, so I bought *The Book of Macrobiotics* in order to know a little something about the subject before I talked to him. Shortly thereafter, I met Michio at the Seventh Inn for dinner and we talked. And it was then that I discovered what kind of person he is, his generosity, his extensive knowledge in every field: anthropology, physics, biology, you name it. I'd never met anyone who had such a wide view of the world. Most of those I meet have specialized themselves so much that they've lost their view of the rest of experience.

EWJ: *When did you meet Michio Kushi?*
Northrup: I met him in March, 1980. I was pregnant at the time and trying to improve my diet without causing harmful effects to my baby. I was worried that if I adopted the standard macrobiotic diet I would bring about all the discharges, the DDT and the rest of the stuff that's stored in the body fat. This would go into the developing baby, and I didn't want that, so I made very gradual changes. I'm still nursing her, and so I've not fully adopted the standard diet for fear that I will be discharging a lot of toxins through my milk. I think very soon though I will start the standard diet.

There's no question that the macrobiotic diet is balanced and provides all the essential nutrients; it answers all the questions, and your intuitive self says this is correct.

EWJ: *Why do you think many doctors today are closed to alternative therapies?*
Northrup: A lot has to do with the medical training we receive. I remember sitting in medical school and hearing the professor explain such and such disease—rheumatoid arthritis, for example—and no one could ever tell you what caused it. The treatments were aspirin and prednisone, which don't cure it. So we didn't know the cause or the cure, but people would come out of medical school incredibly arrogant about what they knew. I kept wondering all the way along, why? We certainly weren't taught to answer a lot of the basic questions that people want to know: Doctor, why do I have this disease? What did I do wrong? How can I cure it?

You're always running into walls. Also, my father told me before going to medical school that when you get your degree the antennas go in and the senders go out. What he meant was that all you do is send signals, and you no longer receive them. Something closes up in you because you are now the authority, and you have gone to an institution where all this knowledge is given out. Information that doesn't come from medical school just isn't valid. And there's a Western prejudice against information coming out of other countries. This prejudice is particularly strong in American medicine; we're a little provincial in this country. If a particular case is studied in France, it's not valid until it is studied in the United States.

EWJ: *Are you observing any change in this attitude today?*
Northrup: Yes, it's wonderful. Many physicians have organized into the American Holistic Medical Association, and this is a terrific support group. It is rapidly growing and trying to study holistic methods, like macrobiotics, scientifically.

But there has been a general and widespread change in many areas of medicine. We live in a world of consumerism now. And in my own field of obstetrics, consumers have changed the field, not physicians. Women don't want to be put to sleep anymore to have their babies. They want to walk around during labor. They pushed to have their husbands present for the birth. When that happened you heard all of the gnashing of teeth, the rending of garments: "Oh, the husbands will disrupt everything. They'll all faint." And you know, I haven't lost a husband yet.

EWJ: *Do you foresee incorporating macrobiotics into your practice?*
Northrup: Yes, I feel it's almost immoral to withhold this information, and this is a conflict that I run into all the time. What if a woman walks into my office with a problem that may be treatable with diet? There's always a part of me that wants to say, "Mrs. Jones, before you take this medication, let me just tell you about this."

As for cancer, we do not have the controlled studies necessary to show that macrobiotics can be effective. This work may soon be in progress, but until we have these studies there is a problem of using macrobiotics with cancer. By the time these people come to the diet they have often had surgery and chemotherapy, and their immune systems are depressed. Then they say macrobiotics didn't cure them, but what possibly could? They were beyond the help of anything at that point.

People—especially some of my colleagues—say to me: "Well, what would you do if you were diagnosed as having cancer?"

There's no question about what I'd do. I would get to the standard macrobiotic diet a whole lot faster.

EWJ: *You seem to be facing a conflict in your life at present between your feelings for macrobiotics and Western medicine.*
Northrup: Oh, yes. There was a pathologist here at the Kushi Institute taking courses recently who told me that she returns to her hospital in Boston every day where she cuts open bodies loaded with cancer and atherosclerosis. And I said to her that there's no turning back once you have this knowledge. There's just no turning back. But I don't think it's that much of a conflict. I have a real network of physicians who are very interested in holistic medicine and in making changes in the present system from within.

I was talking to William Dufty [author of *Sugar Blues* and other works] the other day and he was telling me that twenty years ago everyone thought he was crazy for talking about macrobiotics. But today, his friends are saying that they wish they had done what he did twenty years ago. So there is change.

EWJ: *How do you feel about homebirths?*

Northrup: I have a lot of difficulties supporting homebirths. I would never support legislation, however, restricting someone's right to have the experience, and I do understand how frightened people are about going into a hospital and having their autonomy taken away.

I had the experience of being the doctor for one macrobiotic woman who was going to have a home delivery. She came in for a second opinion. Her midwife had said that she had better go to a doctor, that the homebirth wasn't going to work. She had one of the worst cases of toxemia I've ever seen. Her blood pressure was very high, and I saw her in the clinic that day, and I said to her, "I think we have to deliver your baby now, as soon as possible." She was in a very precarious state. But I could relate to her. I knew what she was trying to do. We started the intravenous and had to use the fetal monitor, but it was okay and she and her husband were very calm about the whole thing and very philosophical. Also, I think they did a great deal for the hospital staff to teach them about macrobiotics. The baby weighed four pounds and was in the intensive care unit. But it was fascinating because the placenta, which should have been calcified and looking like it was unable to nourish the child anymore, was normal looking, only it was small. I even sent it to pathology to have a microscopic section taken. The placenta had none of the changes associated with toxemia. I was fascinated.

EWJ: *What are those changes?*

Northrup: Calcification and narrowing of the vessels. It's almost like atherosclerosis of the placenta. This was one individual case, however, and the great population of macrobiotic women in Boston seem to do very well delivering at home with no problems.

EWJ: *What causes toxemia?*

Northrup: It appears to be associated with protein deficiency, among other things. Tom and Gail Brewer, who wrote the book, *What Every Pregnant Woman Should Know: the Truth about Diet and Drugs in Pregnancy*, have shown this, and Bertha Burk's work in the 1940s at Harvard showed that anyone with lower than 45 grams of protein in her diet per day has a much higher rate of toxemia and stillbirth.

EWJ: *Forty-five grams is the equivalent of what?*

Northrup: Let's see, two cakes of tofu has about twenty grams; it depends upon how big the cakes are. A quart of milk has thirty-two grams; one egg has six grams. A cup of beans has fifteen grams. But every time you combine rice with beans you've increased the amount of protein that's usable by the body. Every time you put gomasio [sesame seeds and sea salt condiment] on brown rice you've increased the usable protein. Soybeans and all soyfoods—such as tempeh and tofu—are very high in protein. It's not difficult to get sufficient amounts.

EWJ: *A small piece of fish contains how much?*
Northrup: Fish is loaded with protein; one ounce of fish has seven grams of protein. So three ounces, which is a very small piece of fish, contains twenty-one grams. I would recommend that macrobiotic women concentrate a bit on getting sufficient amounts of protein. Actually, I would like to do a study to determine how much protein is actually needed by pregnant women. The macrobiotic population here in Boston would be an excellent study group since they often follow a vegetarian regimen that is perhaps lower in protein intake than is generally recommended. The National Research Council suggests that we need an average of about thirty grams and about forty-five grams for the average pregnant woman.

EWJ: *Was the Brewers' study done on an American population?*
Northrup: Yes, it was done in California on a clinic population.

EWJ: *Traditional and Third World cultures, however, get by on much lower amounts of protein in their diets than do Americans. These traditional diets consist mostly of whole grains and vegetables. Is there any data to show that these people might have lower protein needs than Americans?*
Northrup: There probably is data on that, but I'm not aware of it.

EWJ: *What are your general recommendations for pregnant women?*
Northrup: First of all, I like to see a woman and her husband before she's pregnant. And more and more women are coming in to discuss preconception nutrition and health. In general, I tell them that sperm is being produced continuously, but you have all the eggs you're ever going to have at birth. Also, the quality of the sperm can be changed much more easily, so I will often counsel a change in diet with a decrease of processed food and so on. I sometimes encourage someone who is not necessarily predisposed to good diet to take nutritional supplements, because if someone is not going to change their diet then a good multivitamin is of some value. There was a study published in Alaska in 1980 which shows that pre-pregnancy supplementation of the diet with a certain amount of nutrients decreased the level of neural tube defects, for instance when the spinal cord is open and the sac is coming right out the back, or hydrocephalus, waterhead babies. This is an astounding study.

EWJ: *So the first step is to help the person before she becomes pregnant to* *improve her health through better diet?*

Northrup: That's right. And I often counsel to stop smoking because of the devastating effects upon reproduction and to reduce or eliminate coffee and caffeine consumption.

EWJ: *Once the pregnancy takes place, what do you recommend?*

Northrup: I recommend that the woman continue doing what she's doing but include exercises such as prenatal yoga. There are a lot of women who jog. But there are some days when jogging more than two or three miles can be harmful to the baby because it increases body heat and there's no way to dissipate that heat. Pregnant women should really be advised not to use hot tubs. I also advise them to avoid adverse environmental stimuli, for instance, not to read books that are on tragic subjects; to keep the quality of their thoughts high.

EWJ: *Is there any data to support the recommendation that pregnant women should avoid horror movies, for example?*

Northrup: Yes, scientists have found that a frightening movie will cause the fetus to react—totally independently of the mother. Even if the mother is calm and not scared by the film, the baby will nevertheless react. We also know that the baby will move in rhythm with the mother's voice at birth; language is already there, somewhere in the baby's brain, so the baby is extremely sensitive to the mother during pregnancy and is sensitive to what the mother does and says. I think we are finding more and more that there is an individual personality in utero who must be treated as a person who is a passenger but also an integral part of the mother's body. The mother has a direct effect.

EWJ: *Besides protein, what other nutrients do you encourage women to be aware of?*

Northrup: Calcium. A woman can get plenty of calcium by eating green, leafy vegetables like kale and collard greens, sesame seeds, and all sea vegetables. I also recommend a calcium supplement sometimes, made from ground-up oyster shells.

If a woman is not in the mental shape to change her diet, I will recommend milk, though I will say that cow's milk is not the best food in the world. Also, I stress that if they are going to drink milk, they should try to get raw milk from a farm, and in Maine that is still available to some extent. I try to encourage women—if they are going to eat dairy products during pregnancy—to seek out the very best quality.

EWJ: *What are your thoughts on the macrobiotic diet for pregnant women?*

Northrup: For pregnancy the standard macrobiotic diet is fine, but the woman should eat more fish, perhaps, and occasionally some dairy products or chicken. Just the standard macrobiotic diet but a little wider.

EWJ: *This is because of your concern for protein intake?*
Northrup: Yes. Until I get data showing that the protein requirements for pregnant women are less than what I think they are at present, I will continue to recommend that they be concerned about getting adequate amounts of protein.

EWJ: *Beyond that, what other kinds of advice do you give prospective parents?*
Northrup: I just tell them to be in the best health possible and to listen to their bodies. I give them my little talk on circumcision, which I think is an early form of child abuse. The doctor straps the baby down and cuts off the foreskin with no anesthesia. To me it's definitely an abuse of a helpless child. I feel a need to educate parents against this practice. The doctor will tell you that the child doesn't feel it, but any person off the street can see that the child can feel it. I try to stress the sensitivity of the child; many women believe the baby can't see, can't hear. Even Darwin, who observed his own newborn, felt that they were sort of subhuman and that their nervous systems were so poorly developed that they couldn't feel the circumcision. So there's a lot of educating that's necessary to make the parents recognize the sensitivity of their child.

EWJ: *Do you recommend natural childbirth?*
Northrup: Yes, absolutely. You see, the more drugs in the body the more they affect the child during birth. When you use drugs during delivery, the child's sucking reflexes decrease; also the mother is not in a state to appreciate the child and the maternal/infant bonding is hampered. This is a very important thing. Right after the birth of the baby, a period called critical state, the mother is optimally suited to become attached to her newborn. And all the things that a baby does at first to enhance this are dulled by the anesthetics. Sometimes an anesthetic is needed and it doesn't mean a woman can't bond with her child or the father can't bond with the child, but it's definitely decreased. Babies should nurse right after birth; their suckling instinct and reflexes are very strong and this enhances breastfeeding. Studies have shown that the incidence of child abuse is low among mothers who breastfeed and have a good experience the first hour after birth.

One of my big campaigns is to get mothers and babies together in the hospital. Studies have shown that when a mother goat is separated from her kid during the first five minutes after birth, the goat will not accept the kid back. Maternal behavior is distorted. She may not accept it at all. Each species has a specific critical period. Caesarean section mothers have a ten times higher incidence of child abuse than non-Caesarean section mothers.

For humans, this critical period is an hour after birth, because the baby is in a quiet, alert state. The first hour after birth, babies won't cry. They'll be very quiet. They open their eyes immediately if the room is darkened, and they look all around, and they look very old and very wise. They're very awake. They sleep and start to hibernate a few days after delivery, but on that first day, and certainly in that first hour, they're ready to interact with their mother and father.

The problem today is that hospitals are not equipped for this kind of delivery. Most hospitals are set up according to the needs of the forties, not the 1980s. Babies are tucked away in fortresses. Human beings are the only species on earth that routinely and systematically separate the newborn from its mother at birth. And that's another reason why people are afraid of hospitals, because they have just given birth and they're feeling vulnerable; women are in a very emotional state after delivery, and they really can't fight the whole institution, which feels the baby should be observed for a couple of hours somewhere else in the building.

I delivered in Boston at a hospital, but I insisted on having my child with me the whole time and went home in six hours. I think that's ideally what we should have. We should have very safe birthing centers where you are never separated from your child, and you go home very quickly. And even if you don't go home quickly, you should have your baby with you.

EWJ: *When did this critical period start to be cut off between mothers and children?*
Northrup: Since the 1920s, when birthing went into the hospital. But now we're going back the other way, so that most hospitals are giving the baby to the mother on delivery and in the recovery room for that first hour.

EWJ: *Is it true that medicine views childbirth as a sickness that should be treated?*
Northrup: Yes. Up until recently this has been the view among some physicians and only because of the really enlightened doctors is it being changed. Most doctors view pregnancy and childbirth as a disease that needs to be cured. Many experts in the field say that a normal delivery is a retrospective diagnosis, meaning that it's only normal once it's over. And I understand where that view is coming from. We tend to slap a woman in bed, put an IV in her arm, and hook her up to a monitor. When you look at the way birth *should* progress—you should walk around during labor and you should sit up and maybe squat for the

delivery. We interfere a lot with the natural process, so it's almost impossible to tell what a normal birth really is.

EWJ: *When did this current method of giving birth come about?*
Northrup: Well, there are some studies that relate the present method to Louis XIV, who was a voyeur; he liked to watch women deliver, so they were put flat on their backs, and then their feet were put up in stirrups and they delivered this way. But the first woman who stayed in bed during delivery was one of the queens of France. She didn't want to be like the commoners and walk around. She was a patient of Dr. Mauriceau, who was one of those well-known historical figures in obstetrics. I think it was the 1700s; he put her in bed and found delivery went easily this way. He wrote treatises on the subject that were published around the world, and it became common practice to give birth this way. Today, women just accept it from the time they are little girls. They figure that as soon as they go into labor they are going to get into bed. It's a cultural norm. But we now have the data that say that walking around is better and that it shortens labor.

EWJ: *Would you feel comfortable issuing a caution to women who have their births in the hospital?*
Northrup: Yes, I just orchestrated a meeting of nurses and physicians in southern Maine on the subject of giving birth in a hospital, and there was a tremendous show of concern over the issues. The problems involve logistics because the hospitals were built in the forties and now can't meet the needs of the present. But there is a real commitment among many people who work in hospitals to improve the birth experience. At present, I tell my patients about the bonding needs and about breastfeeding. And I also point out that their baby has been in the womb for nine months and ask if it makes sense that suddenly the baby should be put in a room with forty other screaming babies under fluorescent lights in a sterile environment. This is a very shocking environment to say the least. Once you tell people this, many of them want to control their birth experiences. What hospitals need today are birthing centers where the facilities are present to keep the mother and child together.

EWJ: *What are your feelings about the Leboyer method?*
Northrup: He did so much to influence me. I heard him speak and I was very moved. I have incorporated many of the Leboyer techniques in my delivery. There are no lights on in the room, except the one that is right where I'm working. I ask everyone to be quiet, and then we deliver the baby and I immediately put it on the mother's abdomen. I try to think of how this would happen if we didn't interfere. From my

own experience growing up on a farm, I knew that the thing you didn't do when the horse was giving birth was to go into the barn and disturb her. Just leave her alone. So we really have to leave people alone more now with their support people, their husbands, and family. We should just enhance the experience.

However, because of the state of health many people are in today, things can happen, so I want to have the best Western medicine available in the event there is a need for that kind of emergency service.

EWJ: *When do you recommend starting to introduce solid foods?*
Northrup: It's usually about six months, when the baby is beginning to show an interest in solid foods. I strongly urge mothers to nurse their babies for a minimum of six months. If a mother can nurse her child for a year or even two years, it's really great for the child. Of course, we're assuming now that everyone knows that breastfeeding is far superior in every category to formula feeding. It is far superior nutritionally, and it strengthens the bonding between mother and child. Breastmilk is the baby's source of calcium and antibodies; it protects against childhood illnesses, strengthens the immune system, and is living tissue. There's no way formula can duplicate it.

The first food I recommend that the mother introduce is a little brown rice cereal. Mothers should make their own baby food. You can make it yourself in one of those food grinders. It's nutritionally superior to the commercial baby food and much cheaper. I emphasize the cost. Breastfeeding a baby saves you over a thousand dollars a year.

EWJ: *What is your position regarding birth control?*
Northrup: Birth control has been a tremendous factor for change in the status of women, in the whole way they run their lives. But birth control is a tremendously mixed blessing. They've had to take out uteri in women who were only twenty years old because of IUDs and other devices of that sort.

EWJ: *What are your preferences as far as birth control methods are concerned?*
Northrup: First, of course, would be natural methods of birth control. There are many people who use totally natural methods. And that's the ultimate birth control—to know your body, to know when you are ovulating. Then diaphragms and condoms, then last the IUD and the pill, sort of equal, depending on the woman. If she has three kids or two kids already, an IUD is probably a good idea if she doesn't want to think about it. But this is what I want to get away from, the woman who doesn't want to think about the problems associated with the IUD and the pill. This attitude bothers me.

EWJ: *So regardless of the negative effects of the IUD you would still recommend it?*

Northrup: Yes, and I'll put them in in some cases, if that's where the woman's consciousness is right then. Now, I've seen some horrible things from IUDs and they've been associated with many problems including implantation in the uterine wall and increased incidence of tubal pregnancies, but I've also seen women who used them at a certain time of their lives and it was a very good thing for them.

But before I do put in an IUD, I tell the woman the risks that are associated with this device. I sometimes talk about how the IUD may interrupt the flow of energy patterns in their bodies and that we don't know about these things yet, but they are probably there. There's no scientific evidence of energy or ki flow, but I tell them that this may very well exist, and there may be some harm done to that flow of energy with the IUD. I try to be honest, honest to the point that I wonder if I'm not doing a disservice at times because I'm causing more anguish.

EWJ: *You seem to be in a process of transition, and you appear to be changing your ideas on many issues. How do you see yourself ten years from now?*

Northrup: In ten years I think I'll look back on what has had to be done as a necessary evil. I also think that it will be wonderful to be older and wiser. The world will be so changed, and we'll be able to sit back and relax. There's not been any time in my life that I've been able to feel comfortable with the status quo. So someone has to be a catalyst for change. I hope when I'm older to be more enlightened and have a very clear view of the big picture. I want to be living in a different state of consciousness.

EWJ: *So you see yourself as an advocate for a more intuitive understanding?*

Northrup: Yes, I see women in medicine promoting this. There's a wonderful book called *Woman and Nature: The Roaring Inside Her* by Susan Griffin, which talks about women in healing. And women have always brought this intuitive, mothering understanding to medicine, unless the woman has become so male-identified in the medical school or in the male-dominated medical profession that she loses that female instinct. And when that happens, she is like a traitor—you feel betrayed. You go to a female physician for certain reasons. You think you're going to get some different approaches. The woman can provide more of the right-brain, intuitive, holistic approach, and I think that as women we need to trust this. And this is what's happening to women in medicine. Women in medicine will be instrumental in bringing about a more holistic and intuitive healing approach. Also, it's okay if a woman physician wants to hug her patient or show more emotion than what is normally demonstrated. Men are becoming more this way as well. And I see that as good. A lot of medical school students are coming through and are remaining very sensitive. So in the future it will be less of a male/female thing. This is the direction I'm heading in and the direction I see medicine going in, too.

The Motherly Art of Macrobiotics
An Interview with Aveline Kushi

BY BARBARA JACOBS

EWJ: *Aveline, would you please describe some of your personal family history?*

Kushi: I was born in the mountains of Japan about four hours from the seashore by train. I still remember how clean the air was on the top of the mountains. It was so beautiful to watch the changing of the seasons. In the wintertime it was cold and we sometimes had snow. From the time I was about twelve years old, I was so amazed and dedicated to watching the changing of the seasons. I was born in February, in the early part of the spring. That is why when that time comes—the end of February and the start of March—I really love that season. Before anything is starting to grow, it is still under the cold air and clouds and sky and snow and all those things—I really love it. My family was not rich, but we were very peaceful. Our family was Christian. It was so rare for that time—fifty, sixty years ago—in such a tiny town. My parents were the first in town to marry in a Christian ceremony. My father was pretty brave to introduce Christianity, which was rather modern for that time. He also introduced Boy Scouts and Western ways of camping along with some old-style Japanese training to the young boys. I had a total of nine brothers and sisters.

Before I went to Tokyo after World War II, we never used any chemical fertilizer. This way all of our food was natural, organic, and also we had a very large variety of wild grasses and wild plants. We used these in season with other vegetables, and they were so easy to get. The most wonderful memories of my life are of going out into the fields or mountains in the early spring with my mother to pick wild grasses. Those kinds of memories are so strong. Still I can see, I can feel, and smell it all if I close my eyes. And also in the wintertime we would go mushroom hunting. Those things were so wonderful. The water was very delicious. Sometimes we would walk a long way to get special water upstream in the mountains to be used for medicinal teas. Everything was organic, and we never used a gas stove. I never knew of gas stoves until after World War II. We used only wood or charcoal.

It was beautiful.

EWJ: *Were the children in your family ever sick?*
Kushi: Yes. We did not know macrobiotics; we ate meat and sugar, but rarely. In general, because we were poor, our way of eating was good. We tried sometimes to learn the Western style of cooking—but mostly we stuck to the simple, traditional, country-style of cooking. I was eating brown rice before I met Georges Ohsawa. After I became macrobiotic, I just stopped the sugar and animal food, so it wasn't difficult at all for me to change to macrobiotics.

After I finished teachers' college, I was teaching in the mountains, and at that time there was a very famous scholar who was fond of eating brown rice. He was a scholar of classical poems, and these poems I loved very much and that is why I wanted to eat the way he was eating. I asked farmers specially not to polish the brown rice—just husk it. It is so beautiful—just husked rice. It is just like a pearl, a really beautiful small pearl. If you hold it in your hand, it is so sweetly shining.

EWJ: *Can you tell us about how your macrobiotic diet affected your pregnancies?*
Kushi: Once you become pregnant, it is amazing, you change so much. I started to eat much more widely—for me, since before, I was eating very, very simply. Those simple things—vegetables, grains, soups, and sea vegetables—were now not satisfying enough. While pregnant, I sometimes just didn't like brown rice. Or I would have a strong craving for seaweed. Or without thinking, suddenly I would be eating grapefruit. Two or three weeks after the conception of the child, I could feel these cravings. During pregnancy it was sometimes as if a hand would come out of my mouth to take those foods.

It is best not to try control those kinds of feelings during pregnancy but to go with them naturally. If you want to eat something very yin at that time, of course it is better to avoid sugar and chemicals—unnatural things. If you crave yin, try to find some good yin like apples. Also at this time it is good to eat more green vegetables. These are good for the growing child you are carrying.

EWJ: *Can you give us some specific examples of the effects of food on your children or the way you treated any sicknesses they had?*
Kushi: When you are breastfeeding or when you are pregnant, it is easy to control the food the child receives, but after you separate, it is more difficult. In my own case I never had any problems with my children until they began to eat solid food.

I have five children: one daughter (the eldest) and four boys. The girl was a really strong baby, and she had a great appetite. But looking at the total view, I think that since she was a girl I should have given her more yin foods as she was growing up—some Yinnies or fruits which are now so easily available. She was the first, and I was most strict with her diet.

Also, no one was talking about natural foods or macrobiotics almost twenty-three years ago. I had just come from Japan, and I didn't know this country very well. I was only able to get Indian River brown rice and that was it—maybe some oatmeal in the supermarket, also buckwheat groats and some pumpernickel bread. Also, in some Japanese food stores I could get seaweed and buckwheat noodles. Those things were available but nothing else. We could not even get good sea salt. As for tamari and miso, they were unheard of in America then—I was not able to get those things. And, of course, vegetables were not organic at that time. We had only city water.

It was under those kinds of conditions that we were raising children. But my first child was very easy to raise; she didn't have any difficulties. When she was in the first or second grade, I started to experiment with making yeasted breads and I also started to teach macrobiotic cooking. I didn't have any previous experience with making bread, and I thought you had to use yeast to make bread. I didn't know about natural unleavened breads at that time. She was eating these breads and I am sure I used a little too much yeast. I think my cooking was too salty also at that time. You know that Japanese macrobiotic cooking uses almost ten times more salt than American macrobiotic cooking. It was very salty, and naturally, I think, too salty for her. Around that time—I think she was about ten—I found out that she was nearsighted. I was so sorry; it was completely my fault.

EWJ: *That condition was due to too much salt?*
Kushi: I think so. Too much salt creates a great appetite and desire for sweets. Too much salt and sweets puts a strain on the liver, and eye troubles are a sign of liver problems. With macrobiotic children (girls, especially) I think you can give more yin food, less salt than I did—give them a little more variety of yin, especially grain sugar. You can make them natural desserts without refined sugar.

When my children got sick, it was not from yin but from too much yang. When the cooking is very salty and strong (if it's cooked with much fire and for a long time), boys at about ten years old might tend to have some trouble. Muscles get a little too tense. With two of my sons these things came at similar ages. I could see that this sickness was related to some liver and also kidney trouble. One of my sons would become weak and lose his appetite and then feel pain and stiffness all over his body. At first we couldn't figure it out. We asked what he was eating, and he wasn't bingeing much, yet he was very tired. Just a few days before, he was very active, playing baseball with friends, and now he was very tired. At first we gave him tamari and kuzu, but it didn't help. We tried massage and ginger compresses, but nothing changed. I don't know how I figured this out, but I thought maybe I should give some yin. I rushed to the kitchen and grated about three tablespoons of daikon to two cups of water and made a tea for him to drink. As soon as he started to drink it, all the pain and stiffness disappeared very quickly. Then I understood that it was a yang sickness. So I then gave him more green vegetables—cooked a short time—and cooked daikon and raw grated daikon, soft cooked rice, teas, and sometimes apple juice. This same thing happened again when he was going to visit Japan. He was so excited, he became very yang and had the same symptoms; but he didn't want to miss his flight, so he went anyway. Some Japanese took care of him, and he was soon feeling fine.

My fourth child, Phillip, had intestines that were a little weak—I think because in my seventh month of pregnancy I went to Montauk Point at the end of Long Island, a beautiful seashore. It was a very hot summer. At that time I took plenty of fruit, watermelon, pears, etc. I'm not absolutely sure it was because of that, but his intestines were a little weak after he was born. With the other children, I didn't take so much fruit.

EWJ: *What were the symptoms of his weak intestines?*
Kushi: He had a slight hernia. He didn't seem to have any pain. Once in the late fall I put him on a bed near a window, and I was very busy in the kitchen. I think suddenly too much cold came to the baby, and he contracted and his hernia came out—about two inches—and he was crying and crying. He was in so much pain. I had never seen such a thing in my life, and neither had Michio; we didn't know what to do. Without thinking, I went down to the kitchen and grated ginger and made a small cup of tea with bancha, ginger, and tamari. I gave him just a small teaspoon. He only had one or two drops, it just touched his tongue, and the hernia, just like in a speeded-up movie, went back in. He fell asleep peacefully. When he woke up, he was back to normal. All it took was a drop of the ginger. He didn't even have a spoonful! I was so amazed at that time at how effective food can be. Normally in a case like that the baby would be taken to the hospital for an operation. I never studied all these things—about how to treat children's sicknesses—but the treatments just came to me. The hernia was an extreme case, but in small ways, daily, when those things arose, I could judge for myself what to do.

EWJ: *So you think you should learn to trust your own intuition in raising your children?*

Kushi: Of course. One of the most important things to watch is your children's attraction to certain foods. When you put a meal on the table, one takes greens, another wants an apple, another rice—they are all different. I don't have a lot of knowledge about how to treat many kinds of children's sicknesses, just what I learned from Georges Ohsawa's books and teachings—very simple methods.

EWJ: *Often in the fall children have colds, fevers, runny noses. What is the cause of that?*

Kushi: Always there are reasons. You must find out what the child has been eating and figure out the cause.

EWJ: *What about contagious diseases such as measles, mumps, and chicken-pox? When members of a family all come down with the same sickness, could it be because they are eating similar food so their resistance is lower?*

Kushi: They are eating the same food. That is why they usually get sick about the same time. Their condition is similar, so they catch the same things.

EWJ: *How would you treat measles?*

Kushi: Measles is one of the most natural discharges. My children were very healthy and steady when they were babies. I was waiting for them to have measles, so every time they had a little fever I would think maybe it was measles and I would keep them indoors. When they did develop the red spots, I didn't give any baths and didn't take them outdoors. I kept them in a dark, warm room made moist by boiling water on a hot plate for steam. Measles is considered to be a discharge of yang factors from the mother. This explains why we generally treat measles with cooling, dark, humid (yin) factors. Measles usually start out around the eyes and back of the neck and cheeks, and move down all over the body. In the Orient we say that if a child has the measles, he was born yang. Even after the spots are beginning to go away, I keep the child indoors for another week or so, because if measles don't come out on the surface of the skin, the discharge takes place inside the organs and then the baby suffers much more.

EWJ: *How do you deal with a high fever in a child?*

Kushi: If the fever is very high, as in pneumonia or something like that, I get some raw hamburger or carp meat and apply it to the feverish area (for example, the chest). If it is just a cold, a mustard plaster on the chest is good, and it is better not to try to make the fever go down. Unless it is very high, let it run its course.

EWJ: *Do you have any other advice on macrobiotic childraising?*
Kushi: When macrobiotic children begin to have nonmacrobiotic friends, they start to crave sugar. At this time they need some good yin—like naturally prepared apple pies or other good desserts.

EWJ: *I've found that if the natural snacks you make for your children are delicious, your children may even influence their friends by sharing their snacks with them. How do you make sure that your children do not eat too many foods which you feel may not be healthy for them?*
Kushi: If you can show them the relationship between the certain foods they eat and the effects those foods have on them, then they can see for themselves what happens. Explain to them and tell them just to be careful. At this time it is important not to make them afraid of eating different foods, but sensitive to the changes they experience from eating them.

EWJ: *Do you have any advice about weaning?*
Kushi: Macrobiotic mothers generally chew their babies' food for a time after the baby is weaned. I think this practice is good in moderation, especially for hard beans and the like, but the mother's saliva is very strong for the baby, so this shouldn't be done too much or for too long. If you do this all the time, the baby becomes too yang. That is why I suggest that food to be given to a baby should be well mashed but there shouldn't be so much pre-chewing of everything.

Once something is written in a book, the practice seems to become rigid. That is why people have to read with a flexible mind; otherwise mistakes arise. No one writer can explain in written form the one hundred thousand ways of doing things.

For instance, Georges Ohsawa once wrote, ''Do not pick up your baby.'' He was writing to a Japanese audience, where the family is very close and someone will pick up a baby as soon as it starts to cry. He felt this was not so good. In America, on the other hand, many mothers just give the baby a bottle and the baby sleeps in a separate room. In those kinds of situations, it is better to tell the parents to touch the baby, to hold it next to their skin for healing and to develop a warm peaceful type of person. That shows how you must always read written advice with a flexible mind. That is why it is important to be very careful about trying out remedies that you just read about in a book.

EWJ: *Is there anything in particular that a pregnant mother should be aware of, besides her diet, in order to have a healthy baby?*
Kushi: Just as important as food for the pregnant woman is the kind of atmosphere she creates around herself—that she keep herself peaceful. Not that she must be a religious person, but that she have some basic

trust in the order of life, that she not worry—even if she doesn't have money, or a husband. That is one way we can help each other: to encourage each other when pregnant to have a generally peaceful condition. Of course, you may sometimes have an argument with your husband or whatever, but these little quarrels are really happy things. One way to keep a peaceful mind is to meditate—even just for two or three minutes a day. I do this myself.

EWJ: *Is there anything else you would like to add?*
Kushi: Yes. I want to say how grateful to and appreciative I am of my children. They are not perfect, they are not completely strong, they are not necessarily great or geniuses or anything like that, but still they are living their lives. And I am so grateful.

Pregnancy

Diet for a Healthy Pregnancy

BY REBECCA GREENWOOD

Opinions about being pregnant run the gamut from women who use abortion as a form of birth control to those who love nothing more than being pregnant. I am at one end of this spectrum—I love being pregnant! The more attention I give to ovulation, conception, pregnancy, birthing, and parenting the more I am filled with love for life.

Let's examine some of the practical ways to increase our enjoyment of gestation, to properly care for ourselves, and to produce strong, healthy, and happy babies.

If you are pregnant or lactating and new to macrobiotics, I suggest you begin by eliminating extreme substances such as drugs, refined foods, and red flesh foods, as well as possibly reducing your consumption of fruit and dairy products. Otherwise do not be too strict in your eating.

As beginners it is easy to become too rigid and conceptual about your food. If you sit down to supper thinking, "Oh, it's so right to eat this nutritious buckwheat loaf," and yet your whole being is reverberating like a flashing neon sign with the message "PECAN PIE, PECAN PIE, PECAN PIE," for heaven's sake have some pie.

If you continually deny your desires for desserts, sweets, dairy products, and fruits, somewhere in the future you will make balance with something more extreme than an innocent slice of pie. The best way to reduce cravings for sweets and other expansive foods is to reduce your consumption of salt, eggs, fish, and other contractive foods. To achieve balance we must follow the middle path and rely on both our intellect and intuitive messages.

The second pitfall in making the transition to a more wholesome way of eating is to change your diet too quickly. If you were to uproot your favorite African violet, shake all the soil from its roots, and repot it in a different type of soil, what would happen? You would deeply shock it, and likely it wouldn't survive such a harsh transition. Our intestines are our roots. The millions of villi (rootlets) in the small intestine draw nutrients from the food (soil). Both plant rootlets and intestinal villi are skilled at transmuting their familiar environment. Please don't threaten the whole organism with drastic changes. This is especially true if you are pregnant or lactating.

Human cells are composed of nutrients assimilated from food. They contain everything that you've eaten over the last several years—chemical additives and preservatives from restaurant or processed foods, caffeine, novocaine from your last dental visit, nicotine residues, and a fair measure of chocolate and sugar. If you gradually upgrade your diet, the cells composed of the caffeine and novocaine are replaced with rutabagas and barley bread. Normally this is a gentle process, and the more it proceeds, the better you will feel. Sometimes if you dream about, crave, or can almost "taste" coffee, for example, then possibly those cells which were being formed when you were drinking coffee are naturally being broken down, re-entering your bloodstream, and making their way to be eliminated through your body's excretions.

There are numerous ways to quicken the release of these poor-quality cells such as strenuous exercise, sweating, fasting, eating a strict diet, or eating particular foods such as shiitake mushrooms or horseradish. But if you are pregnant or lactating forget the quick ways. For it is your blood that directly nourishes your baby and you do *not* want it full of released toxins. Remember, the guiding rule is moderation. If you want to fast, you have ample time after the baby is weaned to do so. But you might discover that you won't need to fast, for the wondrous thing about creation is that bearing children automatically cleans our system. In the process of generating, we are regenerated.

To many this process of life is miraculous, but unfortunately some women rather than being regenerated relinquish their health. This happened to me after our first child. From sheer ignorance I didn't properly care for myself and my health deteriorated. Fortunately, when I was pregnant with our second child, my husband, Sandy, was apprenticing with a Chinese acupuncturist, Dr. John W. Shen, and we started learning about traditional Oriental medical care during pregnancy and postpartum. Now, several children later, I enjoy better health than before the birth of our first. It was easy for me to trust and follow Dr. Shen's guidance because he was following a tradition that has been effective for 2,000 years and, judging from my husband's stories, he was a master of it. Each day Sandy would come home with stories of how his teacher would know a person's whole health history just from reading his or her pulses. (According to Oriental medicine, there are twelve distinct pulses on the wrists which are palpated to assist in diagnosis.) Here is one such story:

A 45-year-old avid sportswoman, who had enjoyed a healthy and active life, came to the clinic for help. The year before, her health had suddenly deteriorated; she was continuously in severe pain and fast losing her mobility. She went to major hospitals, clinics, and numerous medical experts, but no one knew what caused her suffering or how to alleviate it. Dr. Shen, without talking to her or reading her medical history, palpated her pulses for a few minutes and said: "Soon after delivering your second baby, when you were twenty-eight or twenty-nine, you got a big shock from cold. The cold penetrated deeply, is still inside, and this is causing today's troubles. We'll take the cold out and you'll be fine."

The woman was flabbergasted. He had pinpointed her age with her second baby and helped her recall that in keeping with the modern image of not letting childbirth keep you down, she went skiing within a week after delivery. She remembered that even though she didn't stay long, she got a nasty chill.

Drawing from the traditional wisdom that Dr. Shen and macrobiotics offers, following are suggestions for pregnancy and postpartum to ensure your health and that of your baby.

To begin with, I advise that you create, renew, or strengthen ties with friends of all ages who exercise good common sense. A support system always enriches our lives, but it is especially invaluable during this most vulnerable time. When a well-meaning but misdirected relative sends you newspaper clippings about needing three glasses of milk daily to assure adequate calcium or when your doctor prescribes "harmless" amniocentesis, this is the time to seek support.

Start and end each day by blessing your baby. Offer thanks for this pregnancy, and pray for the baby's health and happiness. I started doing this during my third pregnancy, asking for the baby's health and happiness and imagining a baby who would bring laughter into our family. Asa, now four, is a joyous being with a ready laugh which endears him to everyone. Seeing how powerfully effective my intentions were with Asa, I paid even more attention to my prayers during the last pregnancy. I started with this rather abstract thought: "May our child have health and happiness, and may she develop a great understanding of life through service." As my stomach grew, these thoughts evolved into an unmistakable sense of this baby's unique being and path. At one-and-one-half and still in diapers, Elizabeth has some time to manifest these dreams, but I am still nourished by this prenatal relationship with her.

Pregnancy is a time to fill yourself and your home with order, cleanliness, and beauty. Whatever it is that you've dreamed of— studying flower arranging, taking a needlepoint class—now is the time to pursue it. Find a picture of the Madonna or any mother with child that warms you and hang it in a special place. One of my favorites is a Mary Cassat oil painting which shows just the back of a mother as she arranges a hat on her daughter. Though mundane, it captures the powerful, timeless quality of motherly love.

I also walk a lot, and I encourage you to do the same. Getting away from your household routine and walking is a good time to tune in to your baby and to enjoy fresh air and the beauty around you. Walking, more than any other exercise, helps strengthen and prepare you for an easy delivery. Walking also helps oxygenate the blood, which is important in maintaining an adequate iron level, and it helps your body eliminate toxins. In addition to walking, participate in another form of exercise such as aerobics, dancing, or gardening. Try to use your whole body. Prolonged hours of standing, sitting at a desk or sewing machine, and using only the upper part of your body are best avoided. If you must work while pregnant and if that requires sitting for most of the day, make sure that you frequently get up, move about, and stretch out.

Be it exercise, housework, or sex, do not let any activity exhaust you, as this takes energy from your baby. Don't lift heavy objects for, insofar as possible, you want to keep your energy inward rather than exerting it outward. If you have a two-year-old who is used to being carried, explain that he or she is a big boy or girl and that now you're carrying the new baby all the time. Be firm and persistent, and within a few days your toddler will accept this change.

Keep your kidneys and belly warm at all times. A simple cotton cloth (called *hara maki* by the Japanese) around your middle offers comforting warmth and security. It also softens any harsh noises that otherwise might jar your delicate baby. Silk cummerbunds are a fashionable hara warmer, but their stylish effect might be lost on an eight-month belly. I use a piece of white flannel, 3 yards long and 6 inches wide, wrapped snugly around me, and secured with velcro. It does add a little extra bulk, but it's worth it. Some consider a bikini stunning at any stage of pregnancy. Possibly. For myself, even on warm days, I like to keep my middle covered to prevent the devils from disturbing my energy. Devils?! Now that requires an explanation.

According to Oriental medicine the cause of any disease is from the pernicious influence of one or more of the so-called fourteen "devils." These devils include wind, cold, heat, and excessive emotions such as anger, fear, or grief. To maintain your energy, avoid such extremes. Clothing protects. So don't expose your belly (especially when pregnant) to strong cold, wind, or heat. Try to avoid unpleasant situations such as rush-hour traffic. If in a social situation where someone is expressing anger, pessimism, or negativity, I simply place both my hands over my womb and imagine a protective shield around me, and although I may hear the words, they do not penetrate. I abstain from any movie, book, or TV program which is less than inspiring.

Informing yourself about your baby's growth is another way of tuning in to him or her. Your public library has an excellent selection of books on the subject, and there are fascinating photographs of embryological development. Michio Kushi's chapter on pregnancy in *Natural Healing Through Macrobiotics* (Japan Publications, 1978) is a must for your reading list. He succinctly explains how one day in utero is equivalent to 10 million years of evolutionary development.

Those foods which cool the sexual organs by temporarily restricting blood flow to the uterus are best avoided during pregnancy and the first month of postpartum. They are: raw or sweetened tofu; melons, especially watermelon; any raw food and fruit juices, especially when chilled. Common sense dictates moderation with other foods such as chemicalized or refined foods, frozen or chilled foods, excessive sweeteners, dairy products, fruits, eggs, and flesh foods. But probably the most debilitating of all to your baby's health are: drugs (legal or illegal)—including alcohol, caffeine, and nicotine—and x-rays.

On the other hand, there are foods that are especially good during pregnancy. We can understand why by using the "law of signature" which states: "A food having a quality similar to an organ is good for that organ." Your amazing uterus which is normally a few inches long has such flexibility that it will stretch to 20 inches by full term. We can then deduce that sticky, stretchy foods are good for our sexual organs. Mochi and other sweet rice dishes, natto, and jinenjo are some traditional Oriental foods used for this purpose.

There are other foods that are good for specific problems that may arise during pregnancy. Let's look at some of these.

Calcium

"For every child, a tooth." This old saying is unfortunately based in reality for the many women whose teeth suffer from pregnancy. Your baby needs calcium for his or her developing bones. If you are not ingesting enough, then calcium is drawn from your bones and teeth and carried to your fetus. You can test this by eating sour-tasting foods. Recall how biting into a lemon puts your "teeth on edge"? Sour immediately attracts calcium. Thus if you're craving the classical sour dill pickle, the message behind the pickle is "eat more calcium." You can easily consume enough calcium for both of you and you certainly do not have to lose a single tooth. Natural foods especially high in calcium are all sea vegetables and leafy greens.

Morning Sickness

Morning sickness, as many of us know, is no fun. It is nausea that often occurs in the morning or afternoon during the first trimester. I had it frequently during my first pregnancy. I remember preparing beautiful meals, being so hungry, and yet not able to eat a single bite. I tried various remedies with little or no success. What I finally learned is that an acidic condition causes nausea, and so by my last pregnancies this problem was totally eliminated. To prevent acidity do not overeat, do not eat for two hours before sleeping, and avoid acid-forming foods such as sweets and fruits or even too much whole grain. However, if right now you've got that green glow then try this: Place 1 teaspoon of gomasio (sesame salt) or shoyu (natural soy sauce) in the bottom of a cup and pour hot bancha tea over it. Drink it while hot, take a long walk, and don't eat until the nausea passes.

Toxemia

Toxemia, which is a potentially life-threatening condition, occurs when the white blood cell count is too high. Symptoms include protein in the urine, high blood pressure, swelling in the extremities, and headaches. The standard recommendations are to increase your protein and liquid intake. But the underlying cause of toxemia is not protein deficiency but toxicity or too many impurities in your system. With such a condition your body creates more white blood cells in an effort to clean up the junk. The first step is to stop taking the chemicals and highly refined foods which caused the imbalance. Eat a grain-based diet and your body will naturally regulate this condition. However, toxemia may also occur if you are new to the diet and eating too strictly. If so, by all means widen your diet until after your baby is weaned. If you suspect that you have toxemia, check with your midwife or medical doctor.

Protein

Standard modern medical recommendations are to double your protein intake during pregnancy. Personally, I don't pay much attention to this advice. First, the meat, egg, and dairy lobbies have so exaggerated our need for protein that many of today's degenerative illnesses are caused by the overconsumption of protein from animal sources. Second, your particular protein needs are unique to you. The quantity you need depends upon the quality of the food you ingest and upon how well you are able to assimilate it. If you eat a grain-based diet with daily servings of beans or bean products (such as tempeh or tofu) and if you follow your cravings for dairy products, fish, seeds, and nuts, then you should be consuming ample protein for both you and your developing baby.

Alkaline Urine

Should your midwife be concerned because your urine is slightly alkaline, assure her that it's all right. Most people consume more acidic foods than those eating grains and vegetables, and so the "norm" is for urine to be acid. If your system is slightly alkaline, then a litmus dipped into your urine measures this desirable condition, and you will be less prone to infection, colds, viruses, and other illnesses. Two other ways in which you're apt to differ from the general population is by having a shorter and easier labor and a smaller baby.

Iron Deficiency

During pregnancy a woman's blood supply expands, and so it is normal for her hemoglobin count to be lower than usual. However, don't let it become too low or you'll become anemic, lack energy, and risk excessive bleeding at delivery. To maintain a healthy blood supply eat chlorophyl-rich foods such as dark leafy greens, spirulina, or Green Magma and be sure to get plenty of exercise, especially in the fresh air. Cooking in cast iron pots enriches the iron content of your food. But probably the most concentrated source of iron is sea vegetables. Enjoy seaweed dishes several times daily. Here's a recipe for hiziki condiment; take one tablespoon with every meal and watch your hemoglobin count go up.

Hiziki Condiment
   2 cups hiziki, dry
   water to cover
   1 teaspoon sesame oil
   ½ teaspoon sea salt
Rinse hiziki, then soak it for 5 minutes or until it becomes soft. Drain, and reserve the soaking water. Cut the hiziki into 2 to 3-inch lengths. Heat a cast iron skillet, add the oil, then sauté the hiziki. Add soaking water, then salt, and bring to a simmer. Reduce fire to medium and cook for 1 hour. Add more water if necessary to prevent scorching. Set aside. Now prepare the following:
   2 onions, sliced
   2 lotus roots (or turnips) cut into matchsticks
   2 carrots, cut into matchsticks
   2 burdock roots, cut into matchsticks
   2 teaspoons sesame oil
   ¼ teaspoon sea salt
   shoyu to taste
Heat a cast iron skillet, add oil, and then sauté first the onion, then the lotus, carrots, and burdock. Add salt and then cooked hiziki. Cook covered over a low flame for 45 minutes. Add water if necessary to

prevent burning. Season with shoyu to create a slightly salty, strong taste. Simmer until remaining liquid is absorbed. Serve small amounts as a condiment.

Postpartum

With delivery comes a unique opportunity for you to heal imbalances and to complete the birthing cycle with more energy and vitality than when you started. There's also the possibility that if you don't properly care for yourself, your health may suffer for years. Two different biological phenomena are involved. The first is a hormone called "relaxin" which is produced for the month preceding delivery. As its name implies, it enables you to relax and open up for birthing. After delivery this hormone is no longer produced, but it takes a month for it to leave your system. So for these two months you are biologically (and therefore emotionally and even spiritually) more open and sensitive than normal.

Furthermore, following delivery your body knows not only to produce milk but also to repair your sexual organs. In addition, you can mend not only your uterus but whatever else might ail you, be it chronic sinusitis, lower back pain, or whatever. All that is required of you is to rest and to be nourished with easy-to-digest yet strengthening foods. To accomplish this you'll need the support of your family and friends.

Our Victorian grannies were told that they couldn't walk up or down stairs for the first month. This clever advice kept them upstairs in the bedroom rather than downstairs with the cooking and laundry. Traditional Moslem and Hindu practices dictate that women rest for forty days after delivery. The Chinese and other Orientals suggest a moon cycle or twenty-nine days. According to most of these traditions resting includes not receiving guests, not bathing (except for sponge baths) or shampooing your hair, and staying inside with your baby. During the first week you may get up only to go to the bathroom; the second week and each week slowly increase your mobility until by the end of thirty days you're up and about but still have not participated in normal household routines. By following these guidelines your blood will stay concentrated in your womb and in other areas needing repair. Bathing, shampooing, walking, or doing household chores expends energy outwards and brings blood to the periphery of your body.

Granted, much of this sounds extreme, superstitious, and archaic. But why have so many cultures practiced it for so long? What have you got to lose? Just the postpartum blues.

Once you're a mother, there's no real vacation from caring, nurturing, and being concerned about your children. So how absolutely perfect to take a vacation now. Just you and baby, lying in bed together for days, getting to know and enjoy each other. What a gentle transition for both of you and what an unparalleled opportunity for bonding. Today, most of us are aware of the importance of bonding. My experience is that if this bonding is extended to more than the first few hours, if it stretches into weeks, then your relationship with this baby will be incomparably easier, more joyous, and more intuitive. My month-long bonded babies are more centered and secure. It's a blissful time for both mother and baby.

No matter how good the intentions of a visitor, the energy he or she brings into your home is foreign and takes your energy outward rather than keeping it to yourself and baby. In many traditional cultures, guests do not enter the home of a newborn until after this thirty-day period. Ask your friends and relatives to respect this time for healing and bonding, and welcome them to come and visit after the first month. They'll understand. It is true that grandparents usually *don't* understand (historically, three generations often lived under the same roof), so do make exceptions as appropriate.

Ask a friend or relative to stay for a month to manage the cooking, household, and older children. If that's not possible, have your husband take time off from work, and let the older children stay with grandparents.

The women in our community here in Boulder, Colorado do a round-robin for new mothers who don't have live-in help by taking turns bringing meals for the family. My hunch is that your friends would love to do the same for you.

Foods to favor during postpartum are strengthening ones such as fish soup (made from carp or white-fleshed fish), miso soup, burdock and other root vegetables, simple whole grain dishes, and mochi. During this thirty-day period, try to eat only vegetables and fruit which are cooked. If this seems difficult to do, remember that it is only for a month. Avoid baked pastries, spices, or any other hard-to-digest food. Use enough salt in cooking to give you strength but not so much that you'll want to get out of bed and mow the lawn.

In following the above suggestions, your pregnancy, delivery, and postpartum should be one of the happiest periods of your life.

Dear Barbara

BY BARBARA JACOBS

Q: *I am five months pregnant and my doctor has told me I am anemic. I would rather not take iron pills. Do you have any suggestions on alternate treatments for anemia?*

—Amelia Von Braun
Schenectady, New York

A: Five years ago, when I was about six months pregnant with my first daughter, I was in a similar predicament. I told my doctor that I would like to treat the anemia myself through diet, but that if the results weren't to her satisfaction by the time of my next visit, one month later, I would take iron pills. The next time she checked my blood, she was surprised to see that my hemoglobin count had increased from 11 to 14, but her only comment was, "You must have eaten a lot of eggs." What I did add to my diet were the following:

Tekka

This condiment, consisting mainly of root vegetables, is delicious sprinkled in small amounts over grains or vegetables. It is a very strong, yang food; whenever I use it I notice an increase in energy within one day. About one-quarter teaspoon should be enough if used daily. If you use too much, you may find yourself wanting to drink excessive quantities of orange juice, coffee, or to use vinegar or other acidic foods not particularly conducive to improving your anemic condition.

1 medium burdock root
1 medium lotus root
1 small carrot
1 teaspoon chirimen iriko (little dried fishes)
1½ cups mugi (barley) or genmai (brown rice) miso
⅓ cup sesame oil

Mince vegetables as small as possible. Heat the oil in a cast-iron skillet, and sauté the burdock until the color is light brown and the smell has changed. Then add the chirimen iriko, carrots, and lotus root, cooking each one a little bit before adding the next. Mix in the miso and grated ginger and, reducing the heat, cook for about four to six hours until dry and crumbly. Mix the tekka gently every 15 or 20 minutes to prevent burning. When the tekka is cool, it can be stored at room temperature for many months without spoiling.

Chirimen Iriko

These tiny dried fishes, about the size of small minnows, are available at most oriental food stores. They are rich in iron, calcium, and other minerals. They are a delicious condiment for grains, pasta, or vegetables when dry-roasted or pan-fried in a little sesame oil first.

One of my favorite combinations of chirimen iriko and vegetables is a salad of steamed vegetables and assorted lettuces with a creamy tofu dressing and toasted chirimen iriko sprinkled on top. Soaked, uncooked dulse seaweed is also a tasty and unusual addition to this combination. If you add some cooked elbow or shell macaroni, the resulting noodle salad is a delightful main course for a lunch menu. If your guests are other pregnant women, it is ideal.

Dulse

This seaweed, which is indigenous to the northeastern United States and Canada, is very rich in iron and other minerals. To use as a condiment, first spread it out on a cookie sheet and dry-roast for a few minutes in a 300° oven until it can be crumbled. Then it can be pulverized in a suribachi with roasted sesame seeds (do the dulse first, then add the seeds); this makes a slightly salty, nutty condiment. Of course, dulse can be used in soups, cooked with other vegetables, or simply rinsed well and squeezed out and used in salads such as described above.

Steamed Greens

Dark green and green and white leafy vegetables such as broccoli, kale, watercress, mustard greens, bok choy, dandelion greens, and the tops of daikon radish or carrots are delicious whether used alone or in combination with other vegetables. To prepare any of the above greens except broccoli, place the washed, whole greens in about one-half inch of lightly salted, boiling water. Cover and reduce heat. Remove from the fire after 1 to 5 minutes or slightly more, depending on the size and toughness of the vegetable. The cooking water should be conserved for further use. When the greens have cooled enough to handle, remove excess water from them by holding a handful of greens in one hand over the sink, and squeezing from top to bottom down the length of the vegetable with the other hand. Lay on the cutting board and cut into desired sizes.

Creamy Tofu Dressing

For use with the above vegetables:

   2-3 umeboshi plums (remove pits first), to taste
   one cake tofu, boiled for five minutes
   2 teaspoons sesame oil
   ¼ to ½ cup water, depending on thickness desired.

In a suribachi, combine all ingredients except tofu until they are as smooth as possible. Then add tofu and blend until the whole mixture is creamy.

Greens with Miso

Carrot tops and dandelion or other edible wild greens are also excellent remedies for an anemic condition. One of my favorite ways to prepare these somewhat bitter greens follows:

   2 cups well washed carrot tops or dandelion greens, cut in one-inch pieces
   1 teaspoon sesame oil (dark sesame oil is especially delicious)
   diluted mugi or brown rice miso, to taste
   fresh lemon juice, to taste

Heat the oil in a skillet. Put in the vegetables and, with a high flame, stir lightly and quickly for just about one minute. Reduce heat and add the miso, mixing well to coat the greens. This is easier if the miso is diluted with a little water to a thin consistency. Cover and let cook over a medium fire until the vegetables are tender. Add lemon juice to taste, and remove from heat.

Mochi (recipe below) with mugwort added during the pounding process is also said to be beneficial for an anemic condition.

Red raspberry leaf tea is sometimes taken during pregnancy to facilitate a smooth, fast birth; it is also said to have blood-strengthening properties.

Q: *My first child, now two months old, was born after I had been macrobiotic for about one year. Are there some special foods which I can use to increase my milk supply?*

—Anne Coren
Pittsburgh, Pennsylvania

A: In addition to a balanced macrobiotic diet (i.e., a wide variety of grains, land and sea vegetables, beans, occasional fruits, and small amounts of animal food), there are a few special foods which can be used to improve both the quality and quantity of a mother's milk.

Mochi

Mochi is made from sweet brown rice that has been first cooked, then pounded and steamed. The preparation is somewhat time-consuming, but you can make a lot at one time and store it in a cool place.

A piece of hot mochi in a bowl of miso soup makes a delicious and hearty breakfast on a cold winter morning; and children also love it as a snack with a little rice malt syrup on top. A combination of mochi and steamed greens is excellent for nursing mothers.

5 cups sweet brown rice
5 cups water
6-7 cups sweet brown rice flour

Rinse rice well and soak overnight. Using a pressure cooker, cook at low heat for 40 minutes after the pressure has come up fully. Turn off fire and let the pressure come down by itself.

Remove rice to a large wooden bowl and pound with a wooden mallet, mixing in the flour little by little until it is all well combined. Wet hands in cold water and knead, keeping your hands wet, for about 15 minutes. Bring water to boil in a steamer. Wrap the ball of mochi in a clean damp cloth, and place it on the steamer rack. Cover and steam for about 30 minutes. When you can insert a dry chopstick into the hot mochi and remove it with no mochi adhering to it, the mochi has steamed long enough.

With wet hands, form the hot steamed mochi into three-inch flat rounds. After it has rested about five or six hours it can be baked, pan-fried, deep-fried, or boiled.

Koi-Koku

Koi-Koku is a rich-tasting stew made from carp and burdock root. It is also very yang, so use it sparingly and don't make it too salty. It is so delicious that one easily tends to overindulge, so it is especially important for a nursing mother to use koi-koku in moderation since her diet is directly influencing her child's condition. The following recipe is from *The Chico-San Cookbook,* by Cornellia Aihara.

1 carp
burdock, 3 times the volume (after cutting) as the carp
oil (to sauté burdock)
miso (for a 3-lb. carp approximately ¼ cup)
used bancha tea leaves

Clean the carp and carefully remove its gall bladder, which is very bitter. If you accidentally break it, wash the area immediately with bancha tea. Do not remove the fish scales. Cut the fish into half-inch slices.

Shave the burdock as if you were sharpening a pencil, beginning at the top of the root, and sauté the slices until the strong burdock smell is gone. Add the carp and cover with water.

Put used bancha leaves in a cheesecloth bag. Tie the bag at the top and immerse it in the water with the fish. Bring to a boil and then simmer 4 to 5 hours until the fish bones are soft. Remove the tea bag. Mix miso with a little hot water and add this to the soup. Simmer it one more hour.

If you use a pressure cooker the cooking time is two hours or more, depending on the size of the fish. After letting pressure go down, take out the tea bag and add the miso.

Just before serving, add a pinch of grated ginger.

Note: Use the whole fish, including the head and eyes, removing only the gall bladder. Normally after being caught carp is kept alive in clean water for a day to clean out the intestines. If this was not done, the intestines should be discarded, since carp is a bottom fish and its intestines contain mud.

Seitan

Seitan (See page 165 in the "Natural Lunchbox"), made from wheat gluten, is another food which is good for regaining the strength depleted in childbirth. As with mochi and koi-koku, be careful not to make it too salty.

Barley or whole oats, cooked with enough water to produce a creamy consistency (approximately 5 cups water to 1 cup of grain) are traditionally used in many Western cultures as foods for a nursing mother. Lightly sautéed or Chinese-style stir-fried greens, or lightly steamed greens, are a good balance for the heavier, longer-cooked foods like mochi, koi-koku, and seitan.

There are, of course, methods other than dietary for a new mother to improve her milk. One is to be sure to get enough rest. The first two to four weeks following the birth of the baby should consist of limited activity and no heavy work. The mother should rest as much as possible. This might feel strange to you if you are feeling fairly strong and have a lot of energy, but it has been my experience that if I do too much in the beginning, even light work, I become more tired later. This period of two weeks' rest with no heavy work will be easier for you to maintain if you can arrange to have a friend help you in your home after the birth. After this initial period of about two weeks, you can try to take a nap each day—ideally when the baby is sleeping.

Q: *How do you treat a diaper rash? Also, what kind of soap, if any, do you use to bathe a new baby?*

—Leslie Parker
Reno, Nevada

A: My own children have occasionally had diaper rashes originating from either a yin or yang variation in my diet, during the time I nursed or, in an older baby, comparable changes in his or her own food. In either case diaper rash is caused by an acidic condition. One way to determine whether the cause is excess yin or yang is to observe the quality of the child's bowel movements. If they are greenish (as opposed to mustard-color for a nursing baby or medium brown for a baby eating solid foods), then the cause is probably too much fruit or raw, acid vegetables in the diet (yin). If the stools are very dark and the child seems constipated, there is probably an excess of animal-quality or salty foods in the diet (yang). In these cases, adjusting the mother's and/or the baby's diet accordingly will probably help.

Whenever my children have had to wear disposable diapers for an extended period of time, such as while travelling, they have always had a rash as a result. Another cause is simply leaving the baby too long in wet diapers. A mild rash can be treated relatively quickly and simply by leaving the baby without diapers as much as possible and, in the summer, outdoors. When you diaper the baby, first wash the area with warm water or bancha tea. This will help to neutralize the acidity remaining on the baby's skin from a wet diaper. After the baby's skin has dried in the air, use some cornstarch as baby powder. It's very inexpensive and works as well, if not better than, most commercial products. If the baby has a very dry rash sesame oil is soothing to skin irritations.

I have never used any soap, "natural" or other, for bathing a small baby. They just don't get "dirty." Warm water is usually enough. If you do wish to use something in addition to plain water, make a small bag from cheesecloth and fill it with regular oatmeal or rice polish, called "nuka." This is available from many oriental food stores. The rice polish contains an oil which is helpful to sensitive skin (and is also good for washing the baby's head), and oatmeal is a "fatty" grain, so neither will dry the baby's skin. To make a cheesecloth bag, cut two rectangles of fabric and close up three sides, leaving one short side open. Make a drawstring around the open end, and fill it with the oatmeal or rice polish.

Incidentally, mothers like to have soft skin too, so make a larger one for yourself and you will be pleasantly surprised!

Rx for RH Negative

BY LEONARD JACOBS

Q: *Please comment on the question of Rh negative factors and the possibility of problems with pregnancy.*

—Betty Drake
N. Eastham, Massachusetts

A: Rh is one of the many blood group antigens (substances that stimulate the production of antibodies) found on the surface of red blood cells. Those people possessing this antigen (about 85 percent of the population) are called Rh positive. Those lacking it are called Rh negative. The name Rh came from the Rhesus monkey, which was used in the initial experiments with this antigen. The Rh factor acts as an agglutinogen, which means that it causes a clumping together of red blood cells.

When Rh positive red blood cells enter the bloodstream of an Rh negative person, the recipient may produce Rh antibodies, capable of destroying Rh positive cells. Once an Rh negative individual's blood contains Rh antibodies, these antibodies attack and eliminate Rh positive red blood cells that may enter the stream. If an Rh negative woman's egg is fertilized by a sperm from an Rh positive man, the embryo may inherit the man's Rh factor and its blood will be Rh positive. During the pregnancy or at delivery some of the Rh positive red blood cells may get into the woman's bloodstream. When this occurs, the Rh negative woman may develop antibodies against these Rh positive red blood cells. Once these antibodies are present in the woman's bloodstream, they can pass into the bloodstream of the fetus during a subsequent pregnancy. If the fetus is Rh positive, the Rh antibodies cause hemolytic disease, which results in the destruction of the red blood cells of the fetus in the uterus, causing anemia, heart failure, or other fatal symptoms.

The conventional treatment for the prevention of hemolytic disease is by the injection of the Rh immune globulin, called Rho GAM. This is a specially prepared gamma globulin that contains a concentration of

Rh antibodies. These antibodies suppress the Rh negative mother's immune response to the foreign Rh positive red blood cells that may enter her bloodstream during pregnancy or following delivery. Rho GAM provides practically complete protection by preventing the woman from producing her own permanent Rh antibodies.

The Rh negative mother's blood can easily be checked for the presence of Rh antibodies. The fetus is safe from hemolytic disease as long as the test remains negative. This test is usually performed as soon as pregnancy has been established, and it is generally recommended that it be repeated at least once during pregnancy.

Rho GAM is normally given within three days after delivery of an Rh positive infant. Some doctors feel that administering the Rh immune globulin at between 28 to 30 weeks of pregnancy, as well as after delivery, further decreases the risk of antibody production. However, according to modern medicine women who have already developed Rh antibodies cannot be helped by Rho GAM.

Most doctors feel that unless Rh negative mothers receive Rh immune globulin (Rho GAM), about 13 percent of them will produce Rh antibodies during pregnancy or with the delivery of their first Rh positive child. Women who are not immunized by their first pregnancy have a further 13 percent risk the second time and with each subsequent delivery. So, the more times an Rh negative woman becomes pregnant (from an Rh positive man), the greater her chances are of becoming immunized—of developing Rh antibodies—and having babies likely to have some evidence of hemolytic disease.

According to the macrobiotic approach to health and sickness, the Rh factor is a condition which can be changed by changing your diet and lifestyle. According to this approach, an unbalanced and weak diet will result in the absence of the Rh factor—Rh négative. Eating a diet composed mainly of whole grains, cooked vegetables, beans, and seaweeds, with no refined sugars, red meats, dairy food, or chemicalized foods will ultimately change the Rh factor and lessen the risk of hemolytic disease.

I must emphasize that there is no real proof yet for this hypothesis, and I would not recommend the mother, especially one new to natural foods, to experiment on herself. The theory may hold true for tribal society and longtime macrobiotic women, but in my view it is premature to rely exclusively on diet for this condition. Rho GAM is produced from the plasma of human blood. There seems to be practically no side-effects from the treatment. Therefore, I feel that this immune globulin is advisable for Rh negative mothers soon after they deliver. Of course, a healthy diet can also help, but the risk is quite high if the mother has a second pregnancy but has not had Rho GAM. With Rho GAM, the success is 98 percent.

Birth Control

In Control Birth Control

BY LYNN KAPPLOW

Imagine yourself transported back to a simpler time, when women worked together gathering roots and berries, pounding wild grain, and cooking at an open fire. How do you suppose you would acquire the skills you'd need? You certainly couldn't head to your local bookstore for the latest how-to or sign up for a course at the "Y." Instead you would observe nature at work—the way the plants grew to be just the right taste and color, and how quickly mud dried to secure a hut.

Women probably learned to control conception in a similar manner. They were so in tune with animals that they could sense in advance an animal's coming into heat. When one or two women discovered they too could conceive only on a few special days, they passed this along so that others could regulate pregnancies.

In a most natural way these women were in control. With modern "unnatural" birth control, it is technology that is in control. Instead of expanding our intuition, we reach out to the most mechanical, complicated, impersonal methods. We lie on narrow, papered tables, baring our most intimate parts in our most vulnerable position. This act alone symbolizes our lost control. Bypassing the simple facts of fertility right there within our own cycles, we depend instead on a male-dominated medico-pharmaceutical industry that tends to eliminate, disguise, and distort our own biological rhythm, and separate us from it.

You would think it easy for any woman who so desires to relearn this lost art and get back in touch and in control. But as a teacher of natural birth control, I have found that obstacles arise until the psychological dependency on artificial birth control is faced. My own students have taught me this: Just as a woman's body goes through an adjustment coming off the pill or IUD, just as surely has she suffered pervasive emotional side-effects.

Have you ever thought about the language we use to describe our cycles? Menses (monthly) suggests that all women should have a cycle once a month or risk being considered "irregular" (abnormal). This thinking leaves no room for the incredible variety of individual fertility cycles of women, all normal. Why not, instead, "fertility" cycles? Isn't fertility what our cycles are all about? (As for the "period" portion of our fertility cycle, why don't we just continue to call it our period and leave it at that. Period!) Yes, fertility—as easily distinguished from the remainder of our cycles as are our periods—is a lot more exciting than our periods, and just as visible.

What makes fertility visible is a substance known as "cervical mucus discharge." Why are words like mucus and discharge, ordinarily associated with disease, applied to a natural feminine function? I personally feel uncomfortable with such an unfortunate phrase and much more so when speaking with my students and other women. I'd like to propose instead for this life-affirming substance the term "glide."

Glide is the first of four main indications you can use to recognize your own fertility. As it gently flows from the cervix to the outer vagina you can see it, touch it, and smell it. It glides upon your fingers with a silky, watery feel of its own. It has a distinctive, mildly sweet fragrance. At times it appears cloudy, at times translucent. But the one distinguishing factor is that glide always glistens.

The changes in glide announce the internal progression toward ovulation. At the start of fertility, glide may be cloudy and sticky, but as you near ovulation it becomes translucent and more syrupy and watery.

As soon as ovulation begins glide disappears (though fertility remains). Women usually describe the glide part of the cycle as being wet, based on a general sensation of wetness around the vagina.

During the infertile segment of our cycle, we have a completely opposite phenomenon. Instead of wet, we feel dry, and in place of glide we see nothing. This very nothing is something since it identifies infertility; and within the same phase you can also see a thicker, white substance. Except for the first three dry or "paste" days following ovulation, all the remaining days indicate infertility. And as opposed to the sweet fragrance of glide, the dry and paste days tend to have an acid-to-musty odor.

A second indicator signalling fertility is changes in the cervix, the lower tip of the womb. This tip has a slight opening at the base that protrudes into the upper part of the vaginal canal. It's easily accessible to a touch with the tip of your finger.

As the glide flows the cervix lifts itself higher up toward the womb, creating a roominess in the vagina, and as it rises, the slight opening softens and opens wider. At ovulation it's at its highest, most open position, and immediately following ovulation the cervix closes up and drops back into the vaginal canal.

The third element to warn of approaching ovulation is the body signs. A tingling sensation and tenderness in the breasts and nipples seem to be the most common sign, but others may include an increase of energy, a greater sudden attraction to men, either a decrease or increase in appetite, or a slight backache. Some women feel the actual ovulation itself, a small pinprick sensation in the ovary. Each of us may feel something slightly different. The important thing is to find your own unique sign that repeats cycle after cycle and be alert to it.

The last dramatic change we can notice is the shift in body temperature. Strange as it sounds, women seem to have two normal body temperatures—a low one before ovulation and one at least four-tenths of a degree higher after ovulation. The temperature is the one signal of the four that gives no warning of impending ovulation. Its value is rather in confirming that ovulation has positively occurred.

This peak fertility phase is not all there is to a cycle nor to natural birth control. There are simple techniques for observing day-to-day changes that both lead to and follow ovulation. Women should learn to record their cycles with simple daily charting. Practicing to chart this cycle helps develop confidence.

In my experience, there's something about women studying this topic together that quickly removes barriers and puts women in touch with their own and each other's feelings. It becomes easy in this kind of setting to express honest concerns about themselves and birth control in general. At times during such discussions many women find they're still plagued with lingering emotional scars from previous artificial methods.

Inevitably though, everyone's biggest concern is always, ''What will I do during my fertile phase?'' Let's first consider how long or short a time this may be. On an average, women are fertile for approximately eight days in the entire cycle. However, because each woman is unique and always changing, this average will vary from cycle to cycle. If you plan to prevent pregnancy you need to get in control and make the right choice for those few days. The perfect choice will be determined by your lifestyle and personal beliefs, and choices might change over the years.

For couples who want to continue intercourse during the fertile period there are a few intelligent choices. The pill and IUD are inappropriate since they cannot be combined with this method, both because of their side-effects and their effect on the cycle itself.

Two methods, the condom and the cervical cap, each without foam or spermicide, can be used in combination with this natural method. That's right, *without* foam or spermicide. Both these methods have proved reliable since the 1920s—at least forty years before spermicide. Why not spermicide? Aside from the alarming side-effects, it interferes with glide by masking accurate interpretations or decisions during the fertile phase. I've witnessed many problems among students of mine as well as other friends who've insisted on combining natural methods with spermicides.

The cervical cap is a rubber cap that suctions onto the cervix, creating a tight seal. Rather than leaving the cap in place for weeks I recommend using it as you would a diaphragm: sex in the evening, remove the cap in the morning. This way you continue to observe the changes in the glide as well as receive its benefits to the health of the vagina.

A condom is the simplest of all birth control devices to acquire and if used according to the manufacturer's directions is an effective barrier during the fertile part of the cycle. If your partner puts it on near the beginning of foreplay, you'll have protection from any accidents and consequently you'll feel secure and relaxed.

Some couples practicing natural birth control prefer to forego intercourse entirely during the fertile days. Those who do choose to refrain are surprised to discover a personal inner strength previously unknown to them.

This is a general overview of the natural method of birth control, but you may still be wondering, "Will it work in my individual case?" It will. The method isn't dependent on the type of cycle or situation, it's a total awareness of fertility through any circumstance from puberty to menopause and throughout the entire reproductive years.

In a society supposedly as sexually permissive as ours, I'm always surprised at the large number of sexually inactive women and teenagers attending class. Most find this an ideal time to learn the method, and easily make the transition to active use. Natural birth control is especially useful for teenagers who are not yet sexually active, allowing them to learn the theory of a natural method well in advance of use. This inactive time gives them a chance to build a strong defense against peer pressure. Understanding the facts of fertility dissuades them from believing youthful misconceptions—often the very ones that lead to conception!

What of women at the other end of the spectrum, entering menopause? At this particularly turbulent time, an understanding of how fertility works can clear up much confusion. This is just when women get caught with "change of life" babies. Here, training in natural contraception lets a woman actually see (on her own charts) what's happening regardless of her hormonal and emotional swings, and thereby avoid unwanted pregnancies. The resulting clarity helps her face the reality of diminishing fertility.

Diminished fertility is also experienced by women who nurse on demand. But sometime during the nursing period the baby's needs for food change. The baby becomes less satisfied with breast milk only and seeks more solid food. As these changes occur the mother's body correspondingly adjusts and she may quite suddenly slide back into fertility. But a woman monitoring herself as taught through natural birth control will see those hormonal changes as they shift, receiving early warning signs as fertility approaches and thus avoiding any surprise.

Coming off the pill or IUD can leave a woman with sweeping hormonal imbalances and long-lasting infertility. It's a frustrating time because she wants to return to normalcy but instead will face some unusual and unpredictable changes. All women at one time or another have to handle strong urges to have a baby at any cost. But women coming off artificial methods, often after many years, can be overwhelmed by their sudden outbursts of maternal instinct. They may feel confused, distracted, alternately elated and despondent, and may take unnecessary risks. If this is your situation then it's to your advantage to seek the help of an experienced counselor.

Although we generally think of birth control as preventing pregnancy, the natural method can also be used to achieve pregnancy. Couples learning the method for this purpose are usually worried about infertility. Most find it was only anxiety—and 60 percent conceive within the first three months of practicing the method and 85 percent within one year. Only a small percentage have an infertility problem.

One thought which disturbs many women who've learned of natural birth control is, "Why has this information been kept from us?" We now know, through present-day teachers of this method in remote areas, that the Bantu women of East Africa and Native American Cherokee women openly taught the glide information to their daughters at puberty. It's common knowledge that the temperature coupled with the (ineffective) calendar rhythm method has been around since the 1930s. The use of glide (known as the ovulation method) was developed in the 1950s by Drs. Lyn and John Billings.

One can only surmise that whereas the natural methods don't require expensive materials, ongoing purchases, or office visits, the artificial methods with built-in fittings, check-ups and prescriptions, possible side-effects, and surgical procedures, have been encouraged because of the potential for a billion-dollar industry.

Opponents of the natural method feel the risk of pregnancy may be too high to recommend it, although the journal *Population Reports* lists statistics showing that couples using this method to prevent any births nearly parallel the rate of effectiveness of the diaphragm, and for all users it was only one percent less effective than foams, creams, jellies, and suppositories. It was in the spacing of pregnancies that it seemed less effective. A study done by the World Health Organization in five countries showed the natural methods to be 98 percent effective (WHO, Special Programme of Research, Development and Research Training in Human Reproduction: Seventh Annual Report, Geneva, Nov. 1978). Its study reported that although 97 percent of the women had no problem interpreting their own fertility pattern only 84 percent were effective in preventing pregnancy. It stated that the high pregnancy rates were due to "couples knowingly taking a chance during the fertile phase." Couples who've chosen to disregard the rules and just "take a chance" are making a personal choice which in no way should reflect upon the effectiveness of the methods.

Today because of its growing popularity there's a wide variety of natural birth control methods being taught. They can be learned in a co-ed or women-only group, privately from another couple, in a clinic, from a private teacher, and even through the local archdiocese. You can study glide only or have cervix and temperature included, and learn about foregoing intercourse during fertility or using a barrier.

As you can see there are many choices depending upon your lifestyle. Personally, I feel that the method is best learned in a group with other women. A supportive setting encourages a free exchange of ideas, comments, and criticism, and helps us recognize what we all have to overcome from past methods. In this way each woman will be able to tailor the method to suit her needs, with a responsible decision fully discussed within the group.

In-control birth control, whereby a woman's knowledge of her own fertility pattern is used to control conception, is an ancient new idea—an idea whose time, once again, has come.

The Case Against Vasectomy
This Simple Operation Has Far-Reaching Side-Effects

by LEONARD JACOBS

Q: *What are the effects of a vasectomy or of having the fallopian tubes tied? We have four children and do not want any more but are concerned about the health consequences of any surgery.*

—J. Smith
Philadelphia, Pennsylvania

A: The human body is a unique pattern of biological and neurological interrelationships. Some people also see it as a physical manifestation of electromagnetic or spiritual vibrations, intimately linked to ancestors, children, and the environment. Seeing the body as a pattern of interrelationships is the basis of "holistic" health methods, including macrobiotics. It is a basis for understanding the mechanism of disease and how to treat the whole person rather than only the symptoms. From this perspective, you can examine the question of vasectomy or cutting and tying the fallopian tubes.

These procedures were developed in countries with extreme problems of overpopulation (and for people with serious genetic abnormalities) as forms of sterilization. But these methods of sterilization are seen in most modern societies as practically foolproof ways of enjoying sex without conception. They appear to eliminate the complications of using an IUD or birth control pills, but surgical sterilization has its own side-effects as well.

Since the body is an intrinsically interrelated network, any surgery is going to create an interruption in the biological and neurological flow of energy. The woman's sexual organs manifest the flow of energy spiralling upward through the fallopian tubes to the ovaries. Cutting the tubes will appreciably change that flow of upward energy, which naturally is concentrated in and around the uterus. It often happens that this change will stimulate more intellectual and abstract thinking and a tendency toward more socially extroverted behavior. It is also likely that this surgery will increase the possibility of ovarian and uterine tumors and cysts near the time of menopause.

Vasectomies create a similar disruption in the flow of energy to the man's sexual organs. In this case, the testicles are the end point of downward-spiralling energy. Cutting the channel for the elimination of sperm may produce a tendency toward extreme introspection and narrowness and also the likelihood of infection and eventually cancer.

Surgical sterilization is an extreme procedure that can produce definite side-effects. Natural methods of birth control are not as foolproof but have much less serious drawbacks. Diaphragms and condoms are very effective, and the Billings Ovulation Method involves an awareness of our overall body rhythms. *The Personal Fertility Guide* by Terrie Guay (Harbor Publishing, San Francisco) is an excellent source for learning "how to avoid or achieve pregnancy naturally." It explains how to understand the natural ovulation cycle through observing the woman's basal temperature and cervical mucus which helps the man and woman recognize natural cycles of fertility. *A Cooperative Method of Natural Birth Control* by Margaret Nofziger (The Book Publishing Company, Summertown, Tennessee) is also an excellent guide to natural birth control.

The natural birth control approach helps to deepen our awareness and appreciation of our interrelationship with the environment. Surgery, on the other hand, may make us less sensitive to our natural rhythms and harmony with nature. It definitely changes more than the ability to achieve or cause pregnancy.

Childbirth

Rebirth of Midwives
An Interview with a Practicing Midwife

BY BARBARA JACOBS

I have chosen to have a midwife, Christina Keilt, attend the birth of my fourth child. Christina, who also assisted a physician in the homebirth of my third child, worked as an obstetrical nurse for five years; then, after she had been out of nursing school for about three years and had helped receive her sister's baby, she was inspired to become a midwife. So far(in 1977) she has attended about a hundred births by herself and has assisted in many others.

Christina is a nurse-midwife, which means that she first trained as a nurse, then attended a midwifery school. There are also lay midwives who receive their training through apprenticeship rather than formal education. Some people feel that because birth is a natural process, being a birth attendant is easy, but after attending a few births they realize that it entails more than is at first apparent. Some form of education, either formal or through apprenticeship, is necessary. A new direction in nursing schools that teach midwifery is developing, consisting of a one-year practical experience.

Whatever course of study a prospective midwife chooses to follow demands time and hard work. Being a responsible midwife is a vital and difficult task. Following is an interview with Christina on the rewards and realities of midwifery, and her thoughts and insights on homebirths.

EWJ: *A pregnant woman usually looks for certain characteristics when choosing a doctor for prenatal care and birth assistance. What qualities and qualifications would you suggest a woman look for in choosing a midwife?*
Christina: It's hard for me to say, because it really depends on personal preferences. However, I do think it's an important question for people to think about. Sometimes the assumption is that just because someone is a midwife, she's good. Midwifery currently has a very good name, and in some circles people feel that midwives are better than doctors. Many people also feel that if midwives will do a homebirth they're automatically competent. This is an attitude that should be examined. I'm sure there are some people among the homebirth advocates, or midwives, who just aren't that competent.

I would look for someone who could be a medical guide for me. What I give to my own clients is medical guidance, but I'm not an authoritative kind of figure. Basically what it comes down to is that that person should be knowledgeable, and sensitive enough to allow a woman to create her own birth experience without interference.

Midwifery has become very popular. I could name twenty women I've come in contact with in the past year who have expressed an enthusiastic interest in becoming midwives. But I think it's very important that these people have a consciousness that will go along with what women are asking for—that is, just to be guided in having their own experience and not to be forced into any attendant's particular niche. There's no reason why a woman can't create her own experience, as long as it's medically safe for her, the family, and the baby.

EWJ: *Midwifery seems to require persons who can give a lot of themselves.*
Christina: A midwife can be in a very powerful position. Generally, midwives or birth attendants are respected in a community. But they have to throw away the little bit of power that goes with being good in their work and have humility. As far as I'm concerned, if the birth attendant doesn't have that humility and tries to influence or control the pregnant woman's birth experience, we're just going back to the days of scopolamine and gas. To use that power is disastrous.

EWJ: *What kind of a routine do you follow during prenatal care?*
Christina: The general medical procedures are taking blood pressure regularly, watching the woman's weight gain, checking the healthiness of her tissues, and testing her urine. I observe the growth of the uterus, which really is important, and the baby's heartbeat, size, and position. Another important test is to check the mother's blood periodically, specifically for anemia but also to determine her general health. Another thing I do is talk about nutrition. Of course, this varies with different people, but I think that discussing food intake is very important. Also, just getting to know the person as an individual is very important, too. Sometimes it develops into a friendship, but basically I want to know the mother's likes and dislikes and be familiar with her general lifestyle. She should get to know me too, so when I come to the birth she's not totally surprised at who I am. She'll know what to expect from me.

EWJ: *I remember that, during our initial visit together, you asked why I wanted to have a midwife instead of a doctor. What are some of the reasons women have given you in response to this question?*

Christina: I think the biggest reason is that they're sure I can identify with the birth process more than a man can. Being a woman, I can identify with vaginal and speculum exams, with a baby passing through the vaginal canal. I definitely can empathize with all that. I think another important reason is that my training is different from a physician's. Midwives are trained in the normal. My outlook is that birth is a normal physiological process. Physicians are trained to look at it pathologically. I'm not saying that detrimentally, because physicians can handle pathological problems efficiently, and for that reason I'm really glad they're there. But 95 percent of all births are normal, and a person may want to have someone who is an expert in the normal. I feel that that's what a midwife is recognized for.

Something else that shouldn't be ignored is the financial aspect. Midwives are cheaper, but not because they're second-rate compared to physicians. The reason that I don't charge that much is because I feel that it shouldn't cost so much to do a normal thing. Of course, there should be a fee for the services of people who know what they're doing. But it shouldn't be priced out of people's reach.

Is Circumcision Necessary?
The Risks Outweigh the Benefits

BY BARBARA AND LEONARD JACOBS

If your child is a boy, one of your first considerations is whether or not he should be circumcised. This is a question the parents need to resolve before the baby is born, especially if the child is born in a hospital. Circumcision is now a fairly routine procedure in most hospitals, and unless you have discussed your feelings with the doctor, it's very likely that your child will lose his foreskin immediately after birth (of course, if the parents are Jewish this procedure may be delayed for the necessary eight days).

Circumcision is a fairly old custom practiced by many different cultures throughout the world. The value of continuing this practice has been questioned, and at this point there is no clear consensus among medical practitioners as to its definite value. Historically, there seem to have been two primary reasons for circumcision. The first concerns hygiene: If the young child does not practice regular cleaning under the foreskin there is a possibility of infection. However, if the child's diet does not include many fatty or oily foods, the usual waxy substance that is secreted around the foreskin will not appear, and the problem of infection is unlikely to occur.

The second reason for this custom seems to have come from the need to accelerate the physical and mental development of the newborn. In many cultures that were involved in tribal conflicts or warfare it was discovered that circumcision, which causes early stimulation of the hormonal system, could speed up the maturity of the future male warriors. This is very obvious if you examine the migrating Hebrews and their tribal conflicts at the time of Moses. Many African tribes also seem to practice it out of military necessity.

By removing the foreskin two things happen: The act of surgery immediately stimulates the endocrine system which causes the pituitary gland to begin secreting hormones necessary for growth and mental development; and, once the end of the penis is no longer protected by the foreskin, its constant stimulation will cause these growth hormones to be continually secreted. This essentially means that puberty comes earlier.

There is also a religious reason for continuing to practice circumcision. If you are of the Jewish or Muslim religion (both of which emphasize circumcision), you must decide whether participating in this religious ritual is stronger than your feelings for creating a new set of customs and traditions. It is certainly not necessary to practice circumcision for hygienic reasons, and at this time it also does not seem necessary for the purpose of preparing young soldiers.

Circumcision definitely has its side-effects. In some cases there is extreme hemorrhaging as a result of the surgery. There is certainly some pain involved, but more importantly, it is not a natural practice—if males are born with a foreskin there is no reason to remove it at birth. In the Gospel of Thomas (Chapter 53), when Jesus was asked his opinion of circumcision he replied, "If it were beneficial, their father would beget them already circumcised from their mother." In addition, constant stimulation at the end of the penis, the most sensitive part of this organ, can lead to reduced sensitivity, resulting in a more intellectual and possibly conceptual mentality throughout life. This stimulation increases the child's sensory awareness and leads to an early development of abstract thinking. This was very practical at a time when certain peoples needed to defend themselves against surrounding tribes, but it may result in artificial or somewhat dualistic attitudes toward the natural environment. If we are now attempting to recreate society using natural principles, we may want to consider eliminating this outmoded ritual.

Nursing & Weaning

Mother's Milk

BY BARBARA AND LEONARD JACOBS

The quality of the mother's milk is one of the most important factors in determining a baby's long-term health. Besides eating mochi (pounded sweet rice) and koi-koku (carp soup), there are several other dietary suggestions a mother can follow to ensure that her milk is nourishing.

In examining her milk, the mother's most obvious starting point is taste. If possible, the mother and father should both taste the breast milk, which should be sweet and of a light, milky color. If it tastes slightly acidic or bitter, some modification in the mother's diet is called for. An acidic taste is usually the result of too many raw vegetables, citrus fruits, or refined sugars; a bitter taste may be from too much salt, animal food, or baked food. The other criterion is the baby's condition—if he or she is continually hungry or unable to gain weight, the milk is most likely imbalanced.

A daily diet to ensure nourishing milk could be brown rice mixed with 10 to 20 percent sweet brown rice or barley; steamed hard, leafy green vegetables such as kale, mustard greens, turnip greens, or daikon greens; root vegetables; and miso soup with seaweed. (Make sure that you don't take too much salt or the child will always be hungry and crying.) Cooked fruit and amesake are both excellent desserts to have while nursing. Bancha twig tea and barley tea are satisfying beverages. If you have a problem with the quantity of your milk try to eat more mochi or drink beer without chemicals or additives, such as Guinness Stout, Pilsner-Urquell, or whatever is in your area. If you feel your milk is insufficient in quantity, or you are feeling ill and want to temporarily stop nursing, you might want to find another nursing mother to supplement your milk. The practice of using a "wet nurse" is fairly common in many societies and could be a great help in ours as well.

If your milk is well balanced and nourishing, it should be possible within three or four months after birth to establish a regular nursing and sleeping cycle. An ideal schedule—but one which may only be an ideal—is to nurse every four hours and by the sixth month to have the child sleep all night. During nursing it is important to be calm. This is a good time to read, knit, or do anything that is relaxing and peaceful.

Nursing generally continues until the child either loses interest in milk as a primary food and develops an interest in solid foods, or has several teeth, both of which may happen somewhere between nine and eighteen months. However, the nursing period can be extended for a while longer to postpone ovulation which often works as a natural means of birth control.

As teeth begin to appear, you can bake some hard bread or crackers without any salt to give to the baby to chew on. Homemade hard bread in the shape of small rolls or donuts is easy to hold and chew. Hard, dried fruit such as peaches, pears, or apricots are also good. In addition, during this transition period, you may want to introduce some foods such as soft cooked rice and oats, rice and barley, or rice and sweet rice. Purée it, and sweeten with a small amount of puréed winter squash, rice malt syrup, or amesake. Make the mixture very wet, initially almost the consistency of mother's milk. Since it is puréed, the baby can drink it or take it from a spoon; some pre-cooked kombu (used to make soup stock), or toasted nori may also be given at this time. Continue introducing solid foods to the baby, but until he or she is completely weaned, as a general rule do not use any salt in the cooking of these foods—the baby's digestive system is not developed enough to healthfully process minerals in the form of crystallized salt. However, as the age and stage of weaning varies so much with different children, some may require small amounts of salt and miso before weaning is complete, especially if they are beginning to stand or walk.

Most children will naturally begin eating more and nursing less during the weaning period. Be sure to use a wide variety of foods including green vegetables, sea vegetables, and a small amount of local, seasonal, cooked fruit. This diet should prevent any complications during the weaning period. In the event that the mother's breasts become hard, engorged, or the milk ducts become clogged, apply a mild ginger compress followed by an albi plaster over the sore area. An albi plaster can be easily prepared by grating a small albi or taro potato and mixing it with about 5 percent grated ginger. Place this mixture directly on the skin, cover with cheesecloth and leave for thirty minutes to an hour. If the albi irritates the skin, rub sesame oil on the skin before putting on the albi.

During the weaning period the mother should also reduce the amount of liquid she drinks so the milk eventually dries up.

The Revival of Breastfeeding

BY BARBARA JACOBS

My first exposure to La Leche League was during my first pregnancy when I read the League's basic manual, *The Womanly Art of Breastfeeding*. At that time I had no idea of the League's scope, but after meeting Marian Tompson recently, I was very impressed with the extensive personal attention given to the many League participants throughout the world and the wide variety of information presented in La Leche League publications and classes. This literature is available by mail and covers such topics as the importance of mother's milk and breastfeeding in general, prenatal care and childbirth, childcare, nutrition, and the psychological aspects of breastfeeding. The most recent publication, *The LLLove Story*, documents the history of the League, which was founded in Chicago in 1957. The following interview is the record of a conversation I had with Marian Tompson, former president and founding member of La Leche League, who herself is the mother of seven children.

EWJ: *What is La Leche League?*
Tompson: It's an organization to help mothers who want to breastfeed their babies. We do this through meetings held in homes, literature that we publish, counseling that's available day and night on the telephone and, during the past five years, through seminars for physicians. By attending the seminars, physicians can obtain continuing medical education credits.

EWJ: *Did you personally originate the League?*
Tompson: I'm one of the original group. It began simply as a response to a problem that we as women were having and one which we thought our friends were having, too. I had tried breastfeeding my first three children and had three different doctors with those babies. Each time I ran into what I thought was a problem, with each different doctor the only solution was "put the baby on a bottle." As a result, I never nursed longer than six months with those first three children. Then I met a doctor's wife, Mary White, who had also wanted to nurse and

even though her husband was a physician and very much in favor of breastfeeding, he had absolutely no means by which to help her nurse her first child when she had problems. So by the time we met, I had successfully nursed my fourth child and she had five or six children. We were at a church picnic and of course had our nursing babies with us. Some friends came up and said, "I want to nurse my baby but..." and related the catalog of problems we had also had. It opened our eyes to the fact that other women were having experiences similar to ours. It seemed rather unfair to me that women who wanted to breastfeed had no way of obtaining help, so we decided to hold meetings with our friends who were expecting babies and get together to pool our knowledge about breastfeeding. We contacted five other women who had also breastfed their babies. Mary White's husband, who is a doctor, and his mentor doctor, Dr. Ratner, said that they would be available to help with anything within their area of expertise.

We never intended to become a big organization; we were all busy and happy being mothers and wives. But to our surprise, after just a few meetings women we didn't know came knocking on the door! News of our meetings had spread by word of mouth; we never put notices in the paper or anything. So really, from the beginning it's been like having a tiger by the tail. It's just one of those things, an idea whose time has come; it's just taken off. We've never tried to make it grow or expand.

EWJ: *Why do you think women stopped nursing their children? Is it just an American or European phenomenon, or is it worldwide?*
Tompson: It seems to be happening all over the world, little by little, but probably began here. I think the cause is really a combination of things. One thing is that through pasteurization, milk feeding became safer for infants. Then, when women became suffragists, and started taking jobs and doing more things that men usually did, they could leave their babies with somebody else. But I think the biggest impetus came during World War II when childbirth was moved to the hospital where women were routinely anesthetized and separated from their babies. Also, by that time the formula companies had come into the picture, making their products available. As a result of all these factors, it got to the point where bottlefeeding became the natural thing to do, as far as most women were concerned, and they never even considered breastfeeding. When we started the League we found out that there were a lot of women who wanted to breastfeed and were really bottlefeeding only out of necessity: they didn't know anybody who had succeeded with breastfeeding, or they knew somebody who nursed maybe a couple of weeks and had had to change to bottlefeeding, so they figured why confuse the baby by starting out with

breastfeeding and later changing to the bottle. But as soon as they knew there was a place to get help they were very interested.

EWJ: *What does Dr. Spock say about breastfeeding?*
Tompson: Dr. Spock is somewhat ambivalent. In [the first edition of his book] he said that breastfeeding wasn't very important. Then one time he wrote to me asking for a copy of the La Leche League manual. He said that many women had told him that our book was much more helpful than his. But now, in his regular magazine column, he's come out very strongly in favor of breastfeeding.

EWJ: *Do you have any statistics concerning breastfeeding patterns over the past twenty-one years?*
Tompson: We have statistics from different kinds of studies. I don't know that you can compare one kind of study with another, but there was a study done every ten years in the United States on the number of [new mothers] leaving hospitals who were breastfeeding. The point at which the fewest women were breastfeeding, according to this study, was in 1966 when only 18 percent of [the new mothers] leaving the hospital were breastfeeding. Last year, one of the formula companies who does regular market research surveys said that 38 percent were breastfeeding their babies which means that in ten years it has more than doubled. A recent study [of the readers] of *American Baby* magazine indicated that more than 50 percent of the mothers responding had nursed at least one child.

EWJ: *Is membership in La Leche League growing?*
Tompson: It has grown at such a fast rate we can hardly keep up with it! One way we can gauge growth is by the number of groups we have and how fast new groups are starting. Currently there are about fourteen groups starting each week somewhere in the world, and more than six leaders starting a group every day. Of course this is all volunteer. Last year I think ten new groups started each week.

EWJ: *Are you familiar with any studies that deal with the nutritional value of mother's milk versus cow's milk or formula?*
Tompson: Well, they're basing the formulas on the composition of breastmilk; they are trying to approximate breastmilk. The problem is that our chemistry isn't sophisticated enough to really analyze and isolate all the components of breastmilk at this point. So, as they find things out, they add them to cow's milk. If you really understand chemistry, you realize that the problem is that things work synergistically; you might find through a new chemical analysis that one component of breastmilk is vitamin B6. So you can put that vitamin in, but

there are other things that work with it to make it effective.

EWJ: *That's why they put vitamin D in.*
Tompson: Right, and now we find we don't even need that vitamin D! You see, when we're depending on science to give us the answers, we have to wait until it gets sophisticated enough to give us the answers we need.

It would make sense that human milk has everything needed for a human baby because for millions of years it's been adapted and worked out for human beings. For years it was said, using chemical analysis, that there wasn't enough vitamin D in human milk. Doctors said that this is one thing you have to give the baby. It was usually given in the form of drops, though some more naturally oriented doctors would say to put the baby in the sun. But in the past few months they've said that the reason they thought there wasn't enough vitamin D was that they thought vitamin D was only fat soluble, so they were measuring the amount in the fat portion of the milk, which was only about four percent of the milk. Now they've discovered that there's another kind of and much more vitamin D in the water portion of the milk than in the fat portion. So breastfed babies are getting much more vitamin D than they ever suspected. When you try to analyze something like this you will run into problems until you can analyze it correctly.

EWJ: *Can you give any references for someone who would be interested in more information on research that substantiates the commonsense idea that mother's milk is sufficient?*
Tompson: We have a lot of literature. Derrick Jelliffe has given symposia on the uniqueness of human milk. He has a book coming out in about a month called *Human Milk in the Modern World*, a really definitive book on the subject.

EWJ: *Are there studies relating the psychological and physical development of breastfed children as compared to bottlefed children?*
Tompson: There have been studies done recently, one of them in New York by Alan Cunningham, which show that the morbidity and mortality rates of babies in middle and upper middle class families were considerably lower in babies who were breastfed than in bottlefed babies. This study has just been published in the past year. There have also been studies done in New Zealand and Scotland confirming the same sort of thing. It's hard to measure the psychological aspect. There are some ongoing studies to determine the psychological effect of breastfeeding. It's hard to decide whether a mother who breastfeeds is a different kind of mother—one who has more natural motherliness towards her baby, or how much of it is a result of the mother and baby

interacting together. There were studies done some years ago indicating that children of grammar school age were much more socially adapted if they had been breastfed for a certain length of time. But this is really difficult to measure.

EWJ: *What is your own feeling about the difference between a breastfed and a bottlefed baby?*

Tompson: I think it makes a lot of difference to the mother and to the baby whether the baby is breastfed or bottlefed. I've also heard this from mothers who have bottlefed and then breastfed a baby. They've said, "You never told me how much I would enjoy being a mother." Now, it's important that if you have a job you should enjoy it; your whole attitude toward your work will be different if you enjoy it than if you are doing something just because it's a duty, or because you have to earn money, or whatever. So I think there's an interaction that goes on between a nursing mother and her baby that makes motherhood more enjoyable. The nursing mother secretes a hormone called prolactin that makes her feel more motherly, so even though it's a hard job and involves a lot of time, she doesn't really feel tied down, or like a martyr. Even though people may look at a woman carrying a baby and think, "Oh, that poor girl, she can't put that baby down," actually it's a different thing for that mother. She wouldn't want somebody else to take that baby and go off someplace, she'd feel only half there. So it's something that almost has to be experienced to be appreciated or to know what the difference really is.

EWJ: *What about the father's role?*

Tompson: Good fathering is extremely important. Many mothers couldn't succeed at breastfeeding if they didn't have a husband who was interested in being a good father. Initially, the father's role is not to feed the baby, or even to diaper it or whatever, but to provide stability and support for the mother so she can concentrate on taking care of the baby. He does this in various ways: one way is by financially supporting them if he can, so the mother doesn't have to go out and work. Another thing he can do is fend off the people who might make remarks which could be discouraging and make the mother start questioning what she's doing. He can encourage her by saying that she's doing a good job, and that it's wonderful to see the baby growing on her milk. With this kind of support, she's going to relax, her milk's going to "let down," and her baby will be happy. Thus the father will be contributing in a very important way to the health of that baby. [The "letting down" reflex refers to the spontaneous release of mother's milk whether the baby is present or not. The reflex is stimulated by the baby's sucking but sometimes occurs even when the mother merely thinks about her baby.]

EWJ: *What do you think of the people who say that if a baby is bottlefed the father can play an equal part?*
Tompson: I think mainly that they have a misunderstanding of the father's role. The father is not a substitute mother. He really has a very special role to play, that nobody else can duplicate.

EWJ: *Are there any studies that you know of which correlate breast cancer and failure to breastfeed?*
Tompson: There have been a number of such studies. In fact, one thing I'm working on now in my spare time is setting up a conference on what role breastfeeding might play in preventing breast cancer. The studies done years ago when women were doing what we call long-term unrestricted breastfeeding—that is, not using bottles or solid foods but just breastfeeding their babies—seemed to show quite clearly that breastfeeding helped prevent breast cancer. In fact, even the American Cancer Society used to mention that in their booklet. There's also the psychological aspect which bears directly on the predilection to cancer: Happier feelings are considered to assist in the prevention of cancer and breastfeeding definitely makes the mother happier. But there are other factors, too, such as estrogens, the pill, and environmental conditions which all may have a greater relationship to cancer than does breastfeeding. Birth control pills are known to be related to breast cancer. In fact, you shouldn't be taking birth control pills if you're breastfeeding because it does have an effect on the quality as well as the quantity of the milk.

EWJ: *How reliable do you think breastfeeding can be for birth control?*
Tompson: It's very reliable up to a point. When a baby is being totally breastfed for the first six months—that is, getting all its sucking at the mother's breast and not getting any other food—it's very unusual for a woman's menstruation to return before the end of the first year. Some studies have indicated eleven months as a mean time for ovulation to start. Sometimes a woman will start menstruating, but she may not start ovulating until later. There have been some studies, one which was done years ago through the League, which showed that mothers who relied on breastfeeding had babies slightly farther apart than women who used other methods of birth control. There is a new appreciation of the extent to which breastfeeding does prevent ovulation. Some feel that in the Third World countries where babies are breastfed, this has done more to keep the population down than other programs for birth control. In my own case, I have never ovulated before my menstrual period returned, so once it did I knew that if I

didn't want to become pregnant again, I was going to have to do something about it. I think that's the way it is for most women. There are a small number of women who will ovulate before their first cycle, though.

EWJ: *What would you say about the cost of formula in different parts of the world?*
Tompson: When I was at a congress in India there were many papers presented discussing the cost of formula in the weekly wage of a family. It [sometimes required] 50 percent of the family's wages. Because of the high cost, mothers are watering down the formula and as a result, babies are getting sick and dying. Some years ago, when I was in one of the Caribbean countries as a consultant to the World Health Organization, mothers were asked how long a tin of formula sufficient for four days was lasting, and on the average, it was being used for eleven days. So you can see what weak formula those babies were getting when it was watered down. We know of situations where mothers were just giving their babies water because they had run out of money and were saving up enough money to buy more formula. It sounds incredible to us, but the mothers were convinced by the sales promotion of the formula companies that their babies would be healthier on formula. They weren't being mean or cruel, or even trying to be modern; they were just convinced that it was the best thing they could do, that their babies would grow faster.

EWJ: *Do you feel that these countries are changing mainly because of advertising influences or is the change partly due to the influence of modern medical education?*
Tompson: Well, medical education is a big factor. Many doctors are studying in America and learning a lot about the American way of doing things but not learning about breastfeeding. There is very little, if anything at all, taught about breastfeeding in medical school. This was a real eye-opener at a conference I attended in India: I was swamped by doctors who wanted my advice about how to help mothers with breastfeeding. The doctors believed in breastfeeding, and the mothers wanted to breastfeed, but they weren't succeeding. When I questioned them about their management of breastfeeding mothers, I found they were doing all the wrong things. All the good intentions couldn't change their inadequate training.

EWJ: *Do you have La Leche League chapters in India?*
Tompson: We have a leader applicant in India, but no groups have been formed yet. We have heard from health officials in India who were concerned about what seemed to be a trend toward bottlefeeding,

but no one has applied to be a leader until now. Most of the women who bottlefeed in India live in the cities, and are in the upper classes.

EWJ: *How do you think a mother's diet affects the quality of her milk?*
Tompson: Recently there was a conference in Sweden on that subject. We do know that the kind of food a mother is eating can have an effect on her milk. For one thing, we know the vitamin content of her milk can vary. Some fat levels will also be different. It's really only now beginning to be studied thoroughly.

EWJ: *Of course, as you said before, scientific studies aren't always conclusive.*
Tompson: That's right, they aren't. That's why I think it's a good idea to tell people to eat [according to] their ethnic backgrounds, and eat fresh foods in season which are prepared as naturally as possible. This seems the sanest rule to follow. It can be confusing to base our choice on research, because there's research to substantiate almost anything. I think we usually base our decision on our own individual bias or interest, on what seems right to us and the people who advise us.

They used to say that diet didn't make any difference at all unless the mother had beri-beri, in which case there would be a lack of B vitamins in her milk. Now there are more sophisticated studies, and they're finding some differences from mother to mother. But they're not finding big differences in, for example, the milk of a poor mother and the milk of a middle-class mother. The main differences are in vitamin content.

EWJ: *Do you have a general statement about nutrition? I noticed in your pamphlets you suggest balanced nutrition.*
Tompson: In our manual we tell women to eat a variety of foods in as close to their natural state as possible. Women do get interested in nutrition when they come to La Leche League meetings because they feel that since they started the baby out on the best possible food, they want to follow it with something good. So there's a lot of discussion about food, but not to the extent of learning about different kinds of diets. We do study simple things such as how to read labels (where the mothers can discover how much sugar is in the things they buy) and that natural whole-grain bread is really better than the enriched bread that some agribusiness nutritionists advocate. These are just simple things, but they are steps that help mothers improve their diets, and later, depending on their own particular inclination, they can go deeper into it.

EWJ: *Are you getting more involved in teaching women about diet?*
Tompson: We've been getting more involved in nutritional education at

our conventions and state meetings. The small meetings are primarily concerned with helping mothers to breastfeed; at the larger meetings we have had talks on organic gardening and nutritious meal planning. We also have had several speakers who discussed the diet of pregnant women and lactating mothers. We do try to fill the needs of the people attending the meetings.

EWJ: *What suggestions could you make for a working mother who wants to breastfeed?*
Tompson: We have a booklet for the working mother. Women have always worked, but currently the problem involves the separation of mother and baby. In earlier years, the working mother's baby was with her in the fields, or in another mother's home. The issue is really the separation rather than the nursing of the baby. In the United States I see more women fighting for the right to stay home with their babies for longer periods; they are asking for longer maternity leaves rather than having to go back to work after six weeks. This really wasn't happening very much before many women started breastfeeding their babies. This is what I mean by mothers feeling differently about their babies when they breastfeed them. We are getting a lot of requests from airline stewardesses and teachers asking us to furnish them with material, such as court cases, which show that it's important for a mother to be with her baby. They will use this information to try to get extended leaves of absence. I was just talking to a doctor from Japan, who said that schoolteachers there, if they are breastfeeding, can request up to a one-year leave of absence with the assurance that their jobs will be there for them when they are ready to return to work. This indicates a society that places a high value on good beginnings and close family relationships.

If our society were set up a little differently, the working mother who uses a daycare center would be paid by the government to stay home and take care of her child instead of using that federal money to send the child to the daycare center. In that event, she probably wouldn't even have to go out to work. [In this idealized society] if the mother does have to go to work, she can take the baby. In fact, Margaret Mead said that she felt it was almost more important for a working mother to nurse the baby than a nonworking mother, because that baby has a variety of caretakers and might not be sure who its mother really is. If the mother is not in a situation where she can bring the baby to work with her, she can get a babysitter near her work place, and try to go out at lunchtime and on her coffee break to nurse the baby. If this isn't feasible, she can still just nurse the baby in the morning and at night. Some working mothers nurse a lot during the night. Then she could give the baby either a bottle of breastmilk or formula during the day. I think it is a shame when mothers feel guilty that they have to leave their children to go to work, when the guilt really belongs to society. If our society on the whole felt that mothers and babies were important, these things would be arranged differently.

EWJ: *Do you have any comments to make about natural childbirth and home birth?*

Tompson: I think natural childbirth has a large effect on whether or not a mother is successful in breastfeeding. This is why we talk about childbirth in our meetings. As it happened, all of us who started the League had children naturally, without anesthetics. If the woman and baby are awake after childbirth and the baby is allowed to suck right away, the nursing is going to get off to a much better start, because it has been found that the baby's sucking instinct is most pronounced in the first hour after delivery. If nursing is put off until later, the baby might have trouble learning how to suck. If the mother is awake and able to respond to the baby, this makes a difference too. It's much better to have both mother and baby awake and aware.

As far as home deliveries are concerned, we don't have a standard position but are simply in favor of the mother and baby having the best birth experience possible. It just so happens that out of the seven of us who founded the League, six of us had our babies at home. There are currently eight doctors in the Chicago area who will do home deliveries, but midwives are not legally allowed to deliver at home. I have a great deal of appreciation for the doctor who helped me at home. In fact, all of the doctors in this area who are doing homebirths are fine people.

I think women are more suited to delivering babies however, and one thing that made me aware of this was when my own daughter gave birth at our house. I was there for the delivery, and one friend, a doctor, remarked that deliveries seemed to go more smoothly when there was another woman present who had given birth. A woman's experience makes her sensitive to the moment; she knows intuitively what to do. So I think that in this way, if you have a good, sensitive midwife who has had children herself, you might have an even better homebirth experience. I don't think it's a guarantee, however.

EWJ: *What do you recommend concerning weaning?*

Tompson: This is a very individual matter. Women are so used to bottlefeeding that they think of breastfeeding simply in terms of nutrition. But breastfeeding is more than that, it's a very special kind of close relationship between two people. Everybody has different needs, and you could no more tell a woman how much or how long to nurse her baby than you could tell a husband and wife how many times a day to kiss.

For some babies, this cuddling and closeness and the sucking that goes along with it is needed for a longer period of time than for other babies. I think it's unusual for a baby to wean him or herself totally by one year of age. For some babies the nursing will go on for several years. In the Bible they talk about two years as the minimum weaning age. But our society is so hung up with the sexual use of breasts that people get very nervous about a toddler nursing. I remember a story my mother told me of how, in Italy, a little child would bring a stool to his mother working in the fields so she could sit down and nurse him, and I thought "Oh, is that weird!" until I nursed a three-year-old and didn't think it was weird at all! So it just depends on your personal point of view. But speaking from the child's point of view, it's a perfectly natural, normal thing.

EWJ: *Is there some advice you could give a woman who is weaning her baby but has too much milk?*
Tompson: Well, we do have special meetings just for mothers who are nursing toddlers, because this is a very different situation from a new mother who is coming to a meeting to learn about breastfeeding. But having too much milk for a toddler isn't usually a problem because the milk supply works on supply and demand. If you have a toddler nursing three times a day, that's how much milk you will be producing. The time when there is most likely to be a difference between the amount needed and the amount produced is in the beginning.

EWJ: *If someone were living in a small town or in rural America and wanted information about nursing a baby, how would you suggest she get information?*
Tompson: By writing to us at La Leche League International, 9616 Minneapolis Avenue, Franklin Park, Illinois, 60131, she can find out the address of the group closest to where she lives. We will also send out a free information pamphlet describing our literature. If a mother has specific questions, she is put in touch with a letter writer she can correspond with who could advise her. So, even if a woman is far from an actual group, she is never alone because we'll stay in touch with her as long as she needs us.

EWJ: *What do you see as the trend in breastfeeding over the next twenty years?*
Tompson: I think there will be an increase because people are intelligent and will be more appreciative of how important breastmilk is. I think we will be seeing that the effects of breastfeeding are long-term in the areas of physical as well as psychological health. I also think breastfeeding will spread because as women see how much other mothers enjoy nursing, they will be inspired to try it themselves.

How to Wean Your Child

BY BARBARA JACOBS

T he necessary transition from infancy to childhood takes place through weaning. Breastfeeding is the way a new baby begins life, and after a few months the nursing mother should begin to look for signs of her child's growth toward the next stage of development, that is, increasing independence.

During the time that the baby is in the mother's womb, the only food is mother's blood. Everything the mother eats becomes food for the developing fetus. In the period immediately after birth, the infant is in a transitional stage between the embryonic world of total dependency and the adult world of relative independence. The ideal transitional food in this period is mother's milk. When a baby is nursing, eating only mother's milk, the diet consists of 100 percent animal food.

Since human beings evolved as a result of eating cooked whole grains, the child also evolves into an independent human being with the consumption of cereal grains and vegetable food. Development from infancy to childhood depends on this introduction of vegetable foods. The question is, when?

When the first solid foods are introduced, weaning has begun. In some traditional cultures, such as Native American and Oriental, for instance, many mothers introduce the first solid foods 100 to 110 days after birth (approximately one year from the time of conception), but this rule may not always be advisable or practical. Dr. Spock and most modern pediatricians recommend weaning from breast to bottle by six months (however, it is completely unnecessary ever to replace mother's milk with cow's or goat's milk). The deciding factor in determining when to wean a baby should be the mother's common sense.

Here are three easy clues to look for in determining your baby's readiness to eat solid foods:

1. The baby is not satisfied with milk alone. (It may be that the baby is still too young to be weaned, in which case the problem could be the quality of the mother's milk.)

2. The baby reaches for food when seeing others eat. (Babies with older siblings may do this at an earlier age than first children.)

3. The baby has begun to teethe. This last clue is the most obvious sign of readiness for a change in diet. The timing of this stage may vary quite a bit from child to child (in fact, among my own children, teeth appeared at six months for the eldest and at eleven months for the other two). Teething babies enjoy massaging their gums by chewing on hard, textured things such as a damp washcloth, a piece of carrot (large enough so the baby can hold it but won't be able to break it and choke on it), a piece of hard bread, a dried peach or pear, or a thumb. If you are thinking of cooking some special "teething foods," remember that babies should not eat salt, so prepare the foods without it.

Once you actually make the decision to wean your child, persistence and a sense of humor are necessary. Sometimes the child doesn't seem interested in what solid food is being offered, but don't be discouraged. The extra "little meals" you will be cooking might be exasperating at first, but eventually you will discover what it is that the child enjoys (which is usually what he or she really needs).

When you begin to notice that the baby is nursing more from habit than necessity, you can begin substituting solid foods. At times you may want to nurse your baby for your own convenience, but try to substitute bancha tea or one of the teething foods at these times.

With my first son, I actually made a timetable on which I recorded his sleeping and waking times, his nursing times, and his appetite for nursing. After a week I began to eliminate the "secondary" nursing times (when he wasn't so hungry); then I gradually introduced a meal in place of nursing (for example, when he awoke from a morning nap). I gave him a meal of solids and nursed him afterwards. This way he had his regular nursing, but less milk, and we were both satisfied. The timetable method may be a little tedious, but I found it useful, and it gave me an awareness of the mechanics of weaning which proved helpful with my two other children.

If you stop nursing too suddenly, the abrupt change could be a problem for both you and your child. The baby would miss the close contact, and you might develop engorged breasts. This condition can be somewhat alleviated by ginger compresses and by expressing the milk by hand, but it is extremely uncomfortable and easy to avoid by reducing the nursings gradually. It is easy to circumvent these problems if you remember to take your time; the less the baby nurses, the less milk will be produced. Slow weaning is best, and the complete process can take six months to a year. By the time your baby has two upper and two lower teeth, he or she will probably be more interested in eating solids regularly.

The secondary nursing periods, when the baby isn't so hungry, are often those to which both the child and mother have become most attached. For me, the hardest one to eliminate was the early-morning feeding. Getting up an hour earlier to prepare breakfast instead of conveniently nursing was often a real challenge. I found it was more a problem of weaning myself than weaning the baby. It's all a matter of initiative. When I was finally motivated enough to cook breakfasts regularly, everything else followed very smoothly. The baby would eat breakfast, and the tone was established for the day: solid food before milk. When it seemed that my baby was thirsty rather than hungry, I gave him some bancha tea, using a spoon or cup. (Sometimes I'd mix it with a little bit of apple juice.) Some babies, though they are ready to eat solids at mealtime, might insist on nursing if they see their mother. If this happens, another person can feed and entertain the baby until he or she is distracted from the idea of nursing.

There are three methods of converting cooked food into food that a baby can easily chew and digest. These are prechewing the food yourself to a liquid consistency, puréing or mashing the food, and blending. Food that has been previously chewed by the mother is easiest at first, because the baby's teeth, saliva, and digestive system have not yet fully matured. The baby also does not know how to chew—only how to suck and swallow. Another advantage of prechewing is that you will have food of a correct temperature with no additional heating or cooling. This method is also excellent practice in learning to chew really well. Some people are repelled by the idea of feeding a baby prechewed food, but I always enjoyed chewing my babies' food for them. I felt like a mother bird. Among many traditional people such as American and South Asian Indians, as well as people of our grandparents' generation, prechewing the baby's food was a common practice. If you are weight-conscious, you will be delighted that you are not very hungry after feeding your baby—chewing the baby's food is almost like eating a meal yourself, even though you don't actually swallow much.

Food grinders such as the "Happy Baby" model require repeated fillings since they are very small. When the baby's appetite increases, you will probably want to cook larger quantities of food at one time and purée them in a Foley food mill. (At this time, the baby will probably be ready to eat many of the same foods that adults eat, but remember to set an unsalted portion aside for your child.) I don't recommend using electric blenders as a regular practice, since the enormous vibrational change in suddenly shifting from the most natural way of feeding (nursing) to foods prepared in machines could be quite a shock to a young child. Even if you purée the food in a food mill or blender, in the beginning I suggest prechewing the food as well, in order to mix it with your saliva to begin digestion. When the baby no longer accepts the food from you, let him chew it himself, and remember to continue to encourage the baby to chew. I recommend giving the baby's first foods on a fingertip so that the baby can suck them off, then using a small wooden spoon.

First foods for the nursing baby should be extremely simple and mild. Experimentation is the only way to find out what your child likes best; however, you should consider the season and the origin of the food. Whole grains and locally grown vegetables in season are best in order to help the child stay in harmony with his or her environment.

Many young children enjoy kokkoh, which is a combination of a small amount of beans ground with grains and sesame seeds, and cooked for a long time. Kokkoh not only tastes good, it provides calcium and complete protein. It is also the best way to introduce beans to your baby. Although most young children love to eat whole or puréed beans, they are difficult to digest unless cooked with salt, and will produce gas and discomfort in the baby. When the baby has six to eight teeth and starts to stand up, you may introduce a small amount of whole beans cooked with a bit of washed kombu seaweed to aid digestion. If the baby seems to have a stomachache afterward, it is probably due to inadequate digestion of the beans, so wait for two or three weeks before trying whole beans again.

Nori seaweed is very high in calcium and trace minerals, and a sheet of nori (lightly toasted over an open flame until it changes to a greenish color) is easy for a baby to eat when it is chewed up along with other foods. When the baby is nursing less and has begun to stand up, you may like to try some hiziki, soaked for about a half-hour and cooked with some other vegetables, then puréed. Only a small amount is necessary. Don't be alarmed if the baby has black bowel movements for a day or two after eating seaweed, as this is simply the color of the sea vegetable.

Mother's milk is very sweet, and some babies find the change in taste from breastmilk to solid foods too extreme. To smooth over the transitional period, certain sweeteners may be added to the baby's food. Two whole-grain sweeteners, rice malt and amesake, may be used with a variety of foods. (Both can be made in quantity and stored in the refrigerator, though rice malt, also called "Yinnie syrup," is now widely available in natural foods stores.) One hundred percent barley malt may also be used. Winter squash and carrots, which are very sweet vegetables, can be mixed with cereal or other vegetables (but remember: simple combinations of food are easiest to digest). Apple juice or a little cooked fruit given at the end of a meal is fine for a baby (however, you should be sparing, given too much fruit, the baby may lose interest in vegetables).

Cravings for sweets are usually created by parents, so be aware of the difference between what the child really needs and what you think the child needs. If your child has a persistent runny nose or cries often for no apparent reason, try reducing the amount of fruit and liquid and adding more vegetables. Another way to judge the baby's condition— and to guide your cooking—is to check the baby's bowel movements. If they are very infrequent, or hard and dry, resembling marbles, try using more vegetables with the grains and a little fruit, rice malt, or liquid from simmering dried fruits. In extreme cases, small amounts of maple syrup could be used. Very wet bowel movements can be usually corrected by eliminating fruit and juices, cooking with less water, and making sure the baby's food is well chewed.

Developing your powers of observation and intuition is very important at this stage. Children are so compact and sensitive that any small change in diet has an immediate, noticeable effect.

Mother's milk is the ideal food for an infant, of course, and nursing is a most convenient and enjoyable way to feed a young baby. But the weaning experience can be just as delightful and rewarding for you and your baby, and there's no reason to put off the greatest reward of all: seeing your baby develop into an independent individual with his or her own unique personality.

Teething Bread
   3 cups spring wheat flour
   1 cup corn flour
   2 tablespoons oil
   water
Mix flours, blend in oil, then add enough water to make dough of "ear-lobe" consistency. Knead well (dough should still be soft). Let dough rest in a warm place, covered with a damp cloth, for 2 hours. Shape into loaf, place in bread pan, and bake at 300 degrees until loaf sounds hollow when tapped on the bottom. "Teething rings," of a size that the baby can hold easily, may be formed instead of a loaf; place rings on a cookie sheet and bake.

Oven Toast
   Cut a small amount of unleavened, unsalted whole-grain bread (above) crosswise into ¾" slices. Arrange the slices on a cookie sheet and bake in a 300°F. oven until brown on both sides (turn over when first side is done) and dry inside. When cool, the slices may be stored in a plastic bag and used as needed for teething babies.

Rice Cream Cereal

1 cup brown rice
4 - 6 cups water
1 tablespoon roasted, unhulled sesame seeds (optional)

Rinse brown rice well, then drain and toast in an unoiled frying pan over medium heat, stirring constantly. When rice is a light golden brown and gives off a lightly nutty aroma, remove from frying pan and allow to cool in a wooden or glass bowl. (Some mothers prefer not to roast the rice, which is fine.) When the rice has cooled and the excess moisture has evaporated, grind the rice along with the sesame seeds, as finely or coarsely as you wish, using a grain mill. (Hand-powered grinding is preferred over electric.)

In order to retain their nutritive properties, ground cereals should be cooked immediately after grinding; when exposed to air broken grains begin to oxidize and lose some nutritive qualities. Add water to the cereal gradually and stir continuously to prevent lumps from forming, until it has attained a uniform consistency and begins to boil slightly. Simmer, covered, over a low flame for about 1 hour (or more). A flame tamer helps prevent scorching, as does frequent stirring. Add more water if cereal becomes too thick.

For larger quantities: any cereal that is to be ground may be roasted, cooled, and stored in airtight containers until ready to be ground and cooked. A more efficient method for roasting larger quantities is to spread the grains about ¼ inch deep on a cookie sheet and put them in a 300 degree oven until golden brown and almost entirely dry. Every 20 minutes stir the bottom grains to the top to ensure even roasting. I like to keep on hand an assortment of roasted grains and seeds for use in cereal combinations. Rice, sweet rice, wheat, oats, corn, and sesame and sunflower seeds are good in almost any combination. For children up to six months (or any age with digestive problems), it is better to cook the grains whole, rather than grind them, puréing afterward in a food mill.

Kokkoh

1 cup brown rice
1 cup sweet brown rice
1 cup whole oats (or wheat or barley)
¹/₈ cup aduki beans (or, with wheat, soybeans)
¼ cup roasted, unhulled sesame seeds

Prepare grains and beans as for rice cream. Cook the same as rice cream, using 4 cups water to 1 cup of the kokkoh mixture. Cook over low heat for 1½ to 2 hours (beans take more time to cook than grains).

Vary the types of grains and the proportions. Toasting can be omitted. You can also cook the whole grains and then purée them in a food mill or grain mill.

Some people prefer to use only whole grains and beans in making rice cream cereal or kokkoh. It is thought that flour is difficult to digest for infants, so the same ingredients are used as in kokkoh (or rice cream), but they are cooked whole and then puréed into a soft and smooth cereal.

Soft Rice

1 cup brown rice
8 cups water

Rinse rice well, then simmer over medium-low heat until rice is soft and water is thick and creamy. It is all right if all the water is absorbed by the rice. You can always add more water and cook it a little longer if you want a wetter cereal.

Sweet Juice of Dried Fruits

1 cup dried fruit
2 cups water

Simmer dried fruits (raisins, peaches, or pears) until fruit is tender.

Applesauce

whole apples
water

Core and slice apples and simmer in water, one-half the depth of the apples, until tender (about ½ hour). Purée.

Winter Squash

squash (buttercup and butternut are sweetest)
water

Wash squash but do not peel. Remove seeds and cut squash in 2-inch cubes. Simmer in water one-half the depth of squash. When cooked, the squash can be served puréed or chewed a little, or cut in pieces for older babies who like to eat by themselves.

Rice Malt

4 cups sweet brown rice
7 cups water
4 tablespoons wheat sprouts

Pressure-cook rice in water for 1 hour. Remove from heat and cool to 110 degrees. (Use a candy thermometer for accuracy). At this temperature, the wheat sprouts (ground to a paste in a suribachi) can be mixed in. Maintain the low temperature of 110-120 degrees for 5 hours, if necessary applying very low heat. At the end of this time, press the rice mixture through a cheesecloth to extract the liquid. (The grains are delicious as a base for cookies or "bars.") Cook the liquid, over a low heat, until it becomes syrupy and reaches the desired consistency. The end result should look like honey and taste like butterscotch. (This is homemade "Yinnie syrup," which can also be found ready-made in jars in most natural foods stores.)

Amesake
   1 cup sweet rice
   7 cups water
   ¼ - ½ cup koji rice
Pressure cook sweet rice in 7 cups water for 1 hour. Remove to ceramic or glass bowl (do not use metal) and cool to a temperature that is warm but not boiling hot. (Turn the rice over, so that the rice on the bottom can cool down also.) Stir in koji. Keep mixture covered in a warm, dark place. Stir every couple of hours, and begin tasting after 8 hours to test sweetness. Continue to taste every hour or so until desired sweetness is reached, and then simmer for 20 minutes. If the amesake becomes too fermented, it can still be simmered for ½ hour, which will stop the fermentation and restore sweetness. Purée in a food mill or squeeze through cheesecloth to extract the liquid.

Weaning Your Baby
A Flexible Approach Works Best for Mother and Child

BY PAT SAVAGE

Over the past decade, many parents have begun taking responsibility for their own health as well as their children's. Part of this trend has been the growing popularity of breastfeeding; an increasing number of mothers are attempting to feed their infants in this traditional way. There still exists less than total acceptance of breastfeeding, particularly in public places, but by and large, the sight of a mother with her newborn in the nursing embrace evokes a favorable response.

Yet it seems that no sooner is the breastfeeding relationship established than the inquiries start. "When are you going to start her on food?" or "How long will you nurse him?" may begin as probes from relatives but eventually become concerns that all mothers have to think about. There are wonderful support groups that offer clear advice on the "how to's" of breastfeeding, but there still seems to be somewhat of a cloud surrounding the practical considerations of weaning.

When should weaning start? I am a strong believer in the need for each family to decide what is best. Some nursing mothers must return to work to support their families. There may be other circumstances in which long-term nursing can be a tremendous strain. Whatever the situation, "go slow" is a good rule. Babies seem to make the transition from breast to solids most easily if the substitution is gradual. If the mother will be working full-time, retaining the early morning and evening nursings can smooth out the adjustment for both. Gradual withdrawal from the breast will also help reduce the chance of breast infection as a sudden change in the nursing pattern can cause the milk ducts to become plugged. Should that happen, they can be relieved by baby's nursing or by hand expression.

For our family and for many families that I have known, total breastfeeding—without reliance on bottles, pacifiers, or schedules—has been very rewarding. Breastfeeding helps the baby to make the transition from the womb to the outside world by simulating the prenatal environment of warmth and closeness. The next transition period varies in time for each child. Some mothers sense that their baby is ready to wean when he or she begins walking and taking more of an interest in the world. Others find that the readiness does not come until the third year. In some cultures, the baby is nursed only until he or she is able to live on other foods. Still other societies encourage nursing the child until the age of three or four years or even older. Obviously, cultural expectations play a part in determining when the child will wean.

Even among those who decide on baby-led weaning, there is frequent uncertainty about when that time has come. During a "nursing strike" an otherwise frequently nursing six-month-old, for example, may suddenly refuse to nurse. This can happen during times of illness or exceptional emotional stress. Any child may refuse the breast at any given time, but should the baby repeatedly refuse to nurse over a day or two, it may be advisable to consult with a trained La Leche League counsellor or similarly knowledgeable person. However, your eighteen-month-old who cuts back drastically is not necessarily on a nursing strike.

Another possibility, confusing to first-time mothers especially, may occur when the toddler who has been nursing only a few times a day suddenly wants to nurse as she or he did as an infant. The mother, who is likely to be under pressure from relatives already, begins to panic that her child is going to nurse forever. It is important to keep in mind that for this child the breast is more than a source of nourishment. Since birth it has probably been the child's primary source of pacification and now, when he or she is not feeling well, the child will turn first to nursing for comfort. My experience has been that it's best to go with it on these days. I was, in fact, thankful that we still had this source of comfort to share when my toddler might otherwise have been difficult to appease.

However, it is not uncommon to feel that your toddler is nursing out of boredom. The mother can choose to satisfy this boredom by nursing or with other activities. Every time your baby is satisfied by some other activity, she or he is making strides toward independence. Sometimes a request for breastmilk is actually a request for affection, stimulation, or food. My children both loved books and stories from the first and often their requests for breastmilk meant "I want to sit on your lap and have a story." You are not rejecting your child's need by offering substitutes. Your child will tell you if the substitution is not satisfactory.

Weaning actually starts when the first solid food is introduced. La Leche suggests delaying solids until sometime in the second half of the first year. Usually both mother and child thrive without supplementation for at least six months. Also, your breastmilk is the food designed for your baby, so why not give her or him full advantage? Mothers usually give the baby a cup to grasp at this time, too.

When the baby is ready to eat solids, it depends on both of you whether you want to feed her or him solids first or nurse first at mealtimes. If your baby is in good health or is an older child whom you feel should be eating a substantial amount at mealtimes, it is advisable to nurse after the meal. One of the traps I got into with my daughter when she was a toddler was that she would get cranky and hungry just before dinner. Being caught up in the dinnertime rush, it was easiest to appease her by nursing. She would fill up, and there would be no room for dinner, of course. After dishes were done, she was hungry. Only by making myself slow down at dinner, offering her a nutritious snack before the main meal (e.g., rice puffs, rice cakes, shredded raw vegetables), and perhaps reading a book together were we able to stop the pattern. Once she started eating at mealtimes, both of us showed signs of improved health.

It's not unusual for the breastfeeding child to show plenty of interest in what's happening at the dinner table at a very early age. Particularly at about six months, exploration is an important activity. The baby's interest in food may be an indication of general budding curiosity rather than a "need" for solids. For my son who seemed interested in solids quite early, it was a case of enjoying the sensuous experience of playing with his food. Because he was exceptionally healthy, we decided to give him bits of food when he was about five months old, but he didn't really consume quantities of food until sometime after eighteen months.

Many parents are becoming more and more hesitant about using dairy foods. But even among those on a primarily grain and vegetable diet, it's not unusual to hear concern about what will adequately replace mother's milk. For me, that concern has influenced my bias toward two full years of nursing (until the primary teeth have come in). Common sense must be applied as always, but generally grains such as rice, sweet rice, and oats cooked to a soft consistency are a good starting food. Sweet vegetables such as carrots and winter squash serve to wean baby from sweet breastmilk. Because breastmilk is so sweet and babies are so compact, a little locally grown fruit or diluted fruit juice may eventually seem appropriate. However, my experience has been that a preference for fruits over vegetables can develop if fruit is offered indiscriminately.

I have found that when my children were ready to wean, they responded well to some regulation. Language is a tremendous asset for the older child and discussing expectations concerning frequency of nursing usually invites co-operation, especially if she or he feels part of the decision-making process. With my Katy, we reached a time when she comfortably agreed to three nursings a day, and then we reduced it to once a day at her favorite time. Many children, however, such as my Jamie, taper off quite easily on their own. All eventually do wean, in their own way and in their own time.

The child's needs are one side of the coin. The mother-child relationship is symbiotic; initially baby's needs are more basic and most important. Still, mother's needs and feelings do not operate independently and they are important, too. I feel strongly that it is the quality of the nursing experience that is of greater value than the length of time. Breastfeeding is part of a spirit of total giving. It is common for mothers at some point to have need for some space after the intense devotion of the earliest years. Wherever these feelings come from, they are probably part of nature's plan to assist in the difficult but exciting process of separation.

One of my real tests as a mother has been to learn that no matter what we plan and how much responsibility we want to take for our lives, we do not have ultimate control over them. Another pregnancy, death, illness, or other stresses may change our preconceived notions of how we want to mother. In the event of special circumstances, it may be necessary to hasten the weaning process. If done in the same spirit of love with which the child was nursed, how can it foster other than positive growth?

Weaning is a process that both the mother and the child share and is terminated by the mother's readiness as well as the child's. Although I was quite pleased when my daughter weaned, I have moments when I remember how easy and special nursing was. But the closeness continues with both of my children, now three and six; we all still touch and snuggle. I think there were moments during Katy's second year when we both had doubts about whether there was life after "milky." Today, with her graceful little body on my lap as I sit typing this winter morning, I know most definitely that there is.

Child Development

Making Baby Feel at Home
Your Child Needs Room to Roam and Explore

BY JOANNA AND KOJI YAMAMOTO

Who doesn't feel a kind of wonder upon seeing a newborn baby, and beyond that who doesn't feel a thrill of joy in picking up that baby, holding him close and recognizing he's glad to be with you? After all, it wasn't so very long before—minutes, days, or weeks—that the baby was yet within his mother, absolutely at one with her body, breathing, and mind. For him it feels right to be held, kept close, and directly included in what is going on around him.

But it often happens in the lives of the newborn that they are almost deprived of the strongest sensation they can know—contact! It is as if the cutting of the umbilical cord signals not only the baby's opportunity to breathe and eat with his own body but also to get on in the world as an independent being. He's swiftly carried off for an examination and then deposited in a private box to fend for himself in the experience of emotional deprivation. But isn't it enough to ask him to come out into the world, without having to separate him from significant contact with the mother, his former home and continuing link to survival? Surely, he can't be comfortable alone, and what can he glean from the other babies that might surround him in a nursery, except perhaps that some share a kindred state of isolation?

After the coming of our son, Masashi, onto a futon on the floor of a tatami room in the home of a midwife in Japan, we slept together, him in my arms, for ten hours on the same futon. We have slept together on either our own futon or a mattress on someone else's floor every single night since then. Now, at two years and four months, he goes to his own place in our room and has just begun to sleep through the night without crawling over to me. Masashi never had to overcome the fear of falling from a bed, nor ever had his imagination, body, and mind abruptly halted by the bars of a crib or playpen. Perhaps that is why he is a great and fearless mover. And he never had to cope with going to sleep or waking up consistently with nobody in sight. Perhaps that is why, though such a wee fellow, he is so free—he always speaks first to strangers.

Masashi's birth was quite a happy one, and so it was with all of the babies born in that midwife's home; for even the infants of mothers who could not sleep with them were not put aside. The dear old midwife, at sixty-five years of age and stemming from a long line of midwives on her maternal side, had more than enough of a mother's heart and mind to sleep with the babies herself. Her bed, for all of her midwife life, was next to those babies; and over the years she tended thousands in their first days and nights of life on earth lest they wake up needing someone. She gave me the one essential key to motherhood.

But the experience of birth is not so happy for other babies who number in the millions, the majority, born in American hospitals and relegated to nurseries for periodical checking by masked creatures of hopefully good intentions but perhaps mistaken methods. That isolating mentality is another unnatural product of the scientific atmosphere pervading birth in an American hospital. What happens to the spiritual aspects of a birth muted in a laboratory-like delivery room? It seems that maternity wards manufacture people rather than help mothers let them emerge into this world. Couldn't the room for birth be more similar to the womb: more dark than light, more warm in mood than coolly antiseptic, more natural than metallic in sound, more filled with family than strangers? Birth is like the baby's entry into a new country, but wouldn't all of us be hesitant to disembark in, say, China, to the glare of fluorescent lighting and the sting of metal after a safe and smooth ocean cruise? It is of course a great shock to be born, a shock that can be a most positive awakening into humanity, but to encounter technology at the second of birth seems to be going too far and too fast.

Even at home the process of alienation continues. With dismay I see parents themselves not comprehending the dependent nature and physical needs of a baby. He is confined to his own space, a crib or pen, plus bureau, bathtub, and playthings before he can even see with his eyes let alone hold a toy. He hasn't any idea where he is, except that he's removed. It seems a kind of punishment for having come here.

If security is given through contact, communication, and participation when it is most wanted—from the time of birth to about three years of age—there will be much less adolescent anxiety and creeping existential feelings later on. If the baby is delivered in his own home, or at least in a homey room, by a mother who is awake and not drugged— fully there to first give and then receive him—it is likely that the baby will feel good that he came. And following that, if he is respected at home for what he is—a baby, not a tiny adult—he can do his job of being a baby well enough to give him a good start on doing the jobs of being a child, a teenager, and finally a mature adult.

Breastfeeding is essential for that kind of security, and it seems to work out better if it is not regulated but "on demand." The baby knows when he needs milk or the breast, just as he knows when he's ready to give it up. My son breastfed until he was just a week or so past two, and as we have traveled a lot since his birth, it was really hard for him to let go of the breast—the one sure hold on his base. I talked to him gently about that—how milk is for babies and that he was quite a nice little boy now—and he decided to become a boy. I could see that he pondered it a great deal and really considered the pros and cons of giving up babyhood, but he finally chose in favor of taking on boyhood.

Babies know what they can manage to do or not do and their signs are clear and physical. Just as the umbilical cord stops pulsating and grows dry when it's ready to be cut, so do the baby's neck, hands, spine, teeth, legs, and brain let his parents know when he's ready for holding up his head, holding on, sitting, eating, eating cereal grains, standing, and making choices. He has a rhythm of growth that is his own and if it is imposed upon or made dissonant without consulting him and his rate, it will sound a discordance deep within his nervous system.

These signs assure us that there is wisdom to life, that nature is neither random nor meaningless. The signs are as visible as the oil covering the skin of a just-born baby. The strength of that oil tells us that if the baby were to be born outside in winter he could survive. It is his protection, like a fur coat on an animal, and he deserves to keep it. A baby is not dirty and doesn't need to be soaped. Perhaps some rice bran wrapped in gauze or soft cheesecloth to make a milky suds might be nice at bathtime, but soaps, oils, and even powders shouldn't be necessary, as long as his food is correct.

The signs of a baby's day-to-day health can be felt with your hands and seen in his bowel movements. If when a baby is held under the neck and lower back there is a sense of heaviness that is not merely weight but real solidity and power, he is in good condition. If he feels light or airy, there's some imbalance, usually emotional or physical. If he has diarrhea, warm rice can be put on his navel for up to ten minutes; for constipation you can gently pull and stretch the baby's right leg to stimulate the intestines. If the baby throws up or has a stomach ache, his food or method of feeding is wrong, or his mind is anxious. Is there too much or too little polarity in the home? When a baby is disturbed it is only natural to bring him to your heart where he can find comfort. A warm bath, the mother's heartbeat, and the palms of her hands are the most natural instruments of healing. In any case of distress, the family should simplify their diet, especially the mother, for as long as she is breastfeeding.

Just as the baby exhibits physical signs of his readiness for change and development, so does the body of the new mother. Even if she has been physically active throughout the pregnancy the mother ought to take it easy for some days after the birth, no matter how energetic and elated she might feel with her new motherhood. During the first week, her pelvis is closing, and if her weight is put upon it by walking, it will be strained to return to its normal position. Such strain might later manifest itself as abdominal expansion, dropped organs, incorrect posture, and a tendency to overeat. It's really better for the mother not to walk at all for three to four days or at least until her body temperature is the same under both arms for three consecutive readings. The armpit temperature is directly related to the state of the pelvis, and as each side of the pelvis is closing at a different rate, the temperature will be different under each arm until both sides of the pelvis have closed equally. Then she can get around gradually.

Once the mother is on her feet, she can do some light stretching exercise to stimulate her circulation, but she need not exert herself during the period throughout which she is still bleeding. Then it is best to keep the abdomen wrapped and warm, even in summer, and she really should avoid taking a bath, washing her hair, or doing any kind of work that involves water. Water on the outside cools the body inside, and the pelvis and abdomen need maximum warmth to heal and return to normal. When the bleeding stops, the daily work can be picked up and a program of exercises (such as follows) practiced.

In the first thirteen months after birth, during which the basic portion of the baby's consciousness is being formed, the mother and baby are daily discovering new and interesting aspects of each other. These are, therefore, the most valuable months for securing a mutually trusting, stable, and educational relationship between the parents and child that will enable the child to eventually manage his own life. The baby wants to discover and enjoy the world of his home. Let him follow his curiosity, as his joy is to take it all in. He can be carried with you from room to room, feeling secure in your presence, and be put on the floor, thus freeing his senses to roam and explore. His profession is "growth and expansion" and his techniques are sensation and movement. There is no kindness in frustrating this work. He has lived in the very center of his mother's being for nine months. Surely he needn't now be treated as a caged alien or restricted guest in her home. The baby who feels himself a member of the family—eating, sleeping, looking, listening, moving, feeling, and doing together with Mom and Dad—is likely to be a happy baby in a fortunate home and later on a healthy adult in a peaceful world.

Caring for the Newborn
What To Do When the Baby Arrives

BY BARBARA AND LEONARD JACOBS

T he period immediately following birth is especially important for the baby's long-term health and strength. If the mother has been eating a well-balanced diet and has been doing some regular stretching and strengthening exercises, it is possible that the labor will take between two and six hours, although it may be longer for the first child. However, if an experienced and understanding midwife or other attendant is present and there is a comfortable, secure place for the birth, the labor should be relatively more comfortable even with the first child. The final stage of the delivery will be much easier if the mother hasn't taken drugs or painkillers during labor because she will be conscious and more able to control her pushing and method of delivery. If the labor is long or if there are complications, an episiotomy or the use of forceps may be necessary, but these procedures should not be done routinely just for the convenience of the birth attendant.

When the child is born it's advisable not to clamp the umbilical cord immediately, which is the practice in most hospitals. Since there is about half a pint of blood still in the umbilical cord at birth, it is best to wait until it stops pulsating and turns from pink to a more pale color before clamping and cutting. Cutting the cord early may later lead to respiratory problems or anemia in the child and will also postpone delivery of the placenta.

If the child begins to nurse immediately after the cord is cut, this stimulation will encourage further contractions and the placenta will be immediately discharged. It should be examined to make sure that it is intact. If some part of it is torn, bleeding may occur later on when that part comes out. It is best to save the placenta and bury it somewhere in your garden. Some people think it strengthens the mother to eat it, but this is really not advisable unless the mother is very frail and weak.

If the mother hasn't had any drugs during the birthing process, the baby will usually cry when it feels the colder environment of its new home. This is fine as it strengthens the baby's lungs and helps discharge any mucus still in its mouth or nose. Ideally the mother will be able to keep the baby with her after birth. Allowing the baby to nurse not only stimulates the discharge of the placenta but also helps to tighten the abdominal muscles and contract the uterus back to its normal size. Silver nitrate, which is usually put in the baby's eyes immediately after birth to protect him or her from any venereal diseases the parents may have had, is completely unnecessary if the mother and father have been healthy. If the baby's eyes seem at all cloudy or are filled with mucus, a couple of drops of mother's milk are sufficient to clean them. (The tear ducts in a baby's eyes do not open for several weeks so when the baby cries there will at first be no tears.) Washing off the waxy covering, the vernix, after the birth is also totally unnecessary. You can pat the vernix with a soft baby towel but otherwise leave it to flake off naturally. The vernix, which protected the baby's skin while it was inside the amniotic sack, now offers protection against the harsher environment of air. Washing it off may make the baby more susceptible to skin problems later on.

In the hospital the newborn baby is evaluated by a system developed in 1953 by Virginia Apgar, M.D. The Apgar Score is taken on the new baby one minute after birth. Measurements are made of heart rate, respiratory strength, muscle tone, reflexes, and color. Five minutes after birth a second Apgar Score is taken. These tests are generally useful in a hospital environment, and the mother should know the results. At home, if the pregnancy has been full-term, and if the baby cried, has relatively clear eyes, and can suck, further evaluation is not necessary, though the baby should be weighed to verify that the pregnancy has been full term. The baby should weigh at least 4½ pounds. Anything below that should be brought to the attention of a pediatrician.

During the first twenty-four hours the newborn may not have much of an appetite. This is normal as long as the child begins sucking more vigorously by the second day. During the first two to four days, the mother secretes colostrum from her breasts instead of milk. This clear, sweetish liquid provides the newborn with many antibodies and digestive enzymes and is essential for a strong and healthy child. In the first few days of feeding on colostrum, though, the baby may actually lose a few ounces of weight. This is normal as long as the baby begins to gain weight by the second week.

The fontanelle or soft-spot is another indication of the child's innate vitality. Since the bones in the skull have not totally come together you will see on the top front part of the head a small pulsating spot. This spot will beat with the heartbeat and will seem much more pronounced when the baby cries. The strength of the pulse is an indication of the constitutional strength of the child. The fontanelle should be totally closed and hard by two to two-and-a-half years of age.

Between one and two days after birth the child will have a dark greenish bowel movement called the meconium. This discharge is quite normal and is an indication that the child's intestines are now working properly and that he or she is able to absorb nourishment from the mother's milk. If the child is strong the meconium will be discharged all at one time. Otherwise, it may be several days before it is totally eliminated. After the discharge of the meconium the baby's bowel movements will be yellowish or slightly green depending on the quality of the mother's diet. It will take several months before the bowel movements are more thick and formed and easy to clean off the diapers. As long as the bowel movements are fairly odorless and slightly yellow the child should be in good health.

A common problem during the first few weeks after birth is jaundice. Because the baby's liver is not fully developed until several weeks after he or she begins nursing, some digestive juices, especially bilirubin, may get into the bloodstream, giving the child a yellowish skin color. This condition is very common if the mother has been eating a healthy diet and has been active during pregnancy. In the hospital the doctor may feel alarmed if the baby develops jaundice and may begin testing the bilirubin level by extracting blood from the baby's heels. This test is somewhat painful and in almost all cases is completely unnecessary. Since bilirubin is naturally converted by sunlight to a substance which can be secreted through urination and bowel movements, keep the baby in sunlight for several hours every day. As long as the mother doesn't eat any animal food during this time, the jaundice should clear up within five to seven days. Instead of sunlight, the hospital uses banks of fluorescent lights and keeps the child under the lights for eight to twelve hours each day. This artificial lighting may cause further complications such as fever or diarrhea which may in turn provoke the hospital to do a transfusion, put the child on intravenous feedings, or both. Jaundice is really a natural result of the baby's adjustment to life outside the womb and occurs in almost 40 percent of all newborns.

It is ideal if the mother's activity is light to moderate for at least two weeks after giving birth even though she may feel very energetic. She should get plenty of rest and not get over-tired, but it is important to stay active to maintain good blood circulation during her recovery. Returning to a regular schedule prematurely may result in fatigue or possible hemorrhaging as the uterus heals. Arranging for someone else to do the cooking, cleaning, and other housework allows the mother plenty of time to recuperate and give her full attention to the baby. It is a good idea to continue using some abdominal binding during this recovery period to aid and support the healing muscles which have been stretched during pregnancy. This will also keep the abdominal area warm during the healing process.

The mother's diet after giving birth is also very important. If she tends to overeat or eats large amounts of bread or desserts, it will be difficult for the abdominal wall and muscles to contract to their normal size. If she doesn't eat enough she may become weak and her milk may be less nourishing for the baby. Besides eating a standard macrobiotic diet she can have a bit more steamed vegetables and cooked fruit than usual. Two other strengthening foods for the mother are mochi and koi-koku, as previously discussed. Cooked mochi served with barley malt or rice malt or added directly to miso soup is very strengthening. For producing good quality milk, mochi can be eaten daily during the first several weeks after birth.

The Family Bed
A Loving Human Being Develops from Being Loved

BY PAT SAVAGE

I t is the grey time before the dawn. Before rising, a mother turns to nurse her infant daughter who has stirred. She pulls the baby close to her, catching baby's legs before they nudge her father. On the far side, next to his father, the mother can barely see her son's tousled hair as he continues to sleep undisturbed. These are quiet moments (perhaps the only ones in the day ahead) that mark the passage of darkness into light.

This could be the description of a family on grass mats in a remote African village or on futons in Japan or on a four-poster trundle bed in colonial America. It is, in fact, a picture of my family in rural New Hampshire a few years ago.

In our culture now there is an undercurrent of renewed interest in traditional customs—natural foods, homebirth, breastfeeding, natural family planning. Bringing baby into the parental bed follows in this scheme of things. The trend of separate bedrooms, scheduled infant feeding, bottles, pacifiers, and cribs creates an interruption in nature's plan. Rather than continuing the prenatal pattern of closeness, warmth, and body rhythm, the separation and imposition of adult schedules creates distance. The passage from the womb to the outside world can be smooth if the infant still experiences the warmth and movement that comes from being close to mother. Baby's needs and wants are the same at this time—and what he or she wants is to be held, cuddled, and rocked. Baby's cry has been made to be so irritating for good reason. It sometimes amuses and then saddens me that so much research has been necessary to prove to Western civilization that loving human beings develop from being loved.

Despite mother's and father's intuition, our culture does not offer much support to parents who choose to allow their children to sleep with them. With the taboo that exists, many parents hesitate to act on their deeper feelings that baby's need for closeness does not cease at night. And for that reason it is helpful to be able to look at some research. Far from being a new concept, the family bed has its roots in both primitive and civilized cultures.

One anthropologist studied fifty-six societies and found that in forty-eight of them, babies and mothers slept together for at least the first year of life. In about half these cultures baby was between the mother and father. In another study of 186 cultures, the baby was always in the same room with the mother, although the father in some groups slept in another room. It appears that some cultures recognize the change in the mother's focus with the child's arrival and that in these cultures the marital bed is not the sanctimonious institution it has become in ours.

Cross-cultural observation offers many examples of co-family sleeping. In Bali, for instance, the child is always in close physical contact with someone and everyone sleeps together. The *Family Bed* by Tine Thevenin includes accounts by missionaries, anthropologists, and doctors that show the happy effects developing from family closeness. In a Philippino family, the youngest child slept with its parents, and the older six children slept with each other. A Peace Corps volunteer who lived with them for two years never observed them quarreling. Eskimos who sleep together have often been observed to be happy and well-integrated as both children and adults. The warm and convivial environment they create for themselves surely has survival value in their extremely cold climate.

Margaret Mead made a provocative study of two different South Sea tribes, the Arapesh and the Mundugumor. The Arapesh are typified by amicability, love, and trust. Their childrearing practices manifest their great love of children and include constant physical contact, breastfeeding on demand, and baby-led weaning. The other tribe, the Mundugumor, are hateful and distrustful. Pregnancy and childrearing are the lowest of occupations. They breastfeed their babies only when they will not stop crying and only until they can survive on other foods.

Western history also offers support for the custom of co-family sleeping. One-hundred-fifty years ago, sleeping quarters were frequently shared by all (and in some places they still are). Bedding would often be seen in an area where there was a lot of other activity, for example, in the kitchen. While particularly true among the peasantry, this failure to associate privacy, separation, and sexual taboo with the bedroom was not limited to any one class: The English Royal Family had a bed that could sleep 102 persons; Louis XVI often conducted *affaires d'etat* from his luxurious canopied bed.

The trinity bed, an English invention, was brought to America and enjoyed popularity here as the "trundle bed," a family bed with two "drawers" that pulled out from underneath. While it varied depending on a family's needs, the top bed was usually reserved for family members and the "drawers" for the servants.

The custom of bundling—a man and a woman clothed and lying on the same bed—was practiced here in America during the later eighteenth century. Even the Puritans allowed this practice. Martha Washington's diary and letters to George casually refer to male friends with whom she spent cold, damp winter evenings chatting away under the bed covers. Perhaps space considerations and lack of central heating were the most important factors in determining sleeping arrangements in the past, but these images give our present consciousness grounding. What is important is that co-family sleeping is a traditional custom that can help to meet needs that are unchanging with time.

Ideological considerations aside, what is it like to sleep in the family bed? It was almost effortless for us to keep both of our children in bed with us in their early infancies. Other than the satisfaction of knowing that you are serving the children's needs best, the whole family feels great joy in waking up together. Having a few moments of cuddling and horseplay is a good way to start the day before each member goes his or her own way.

And it seems that nature meant for mothers and babies to sleep together in order to assure a good night's sleep for both. When our son was a round-the-clock breastfeeder, it was very easy to bring him to bed with us. When asked how often I nursed my baby at night, I honestly could not say. Rolling over to nurse became instinctive and our sleep was rarely interrupted. The common picture of restless nights with mother waking to prepare for the 2:00 A.M. feeding was one we were able to avoid. However, what is natural is not always what is easy. Babies do grow in size and often change their sleeping patterns as well as sleeping positions. Our children have gone through a variety of changes. There have been periods when we would wake during the night to find the baby sleeping horizontally between us or crouched between pillows at the head of the bed. We adjusted to each new challenging position and found persistence and a sense of humor invaluable aids.

New parents who feel right about having their infant between them in bed often have questions about just how long they can expect he or she will want to be there. Every child is different and develops autonomy at its own pace. My children responded well to having their own sleeping space around the time they were weaning and toilet training, a little before the third year. Motivated by my second pregnancy, we "weaned" Jamie to his own mattress in our room. While he still enjoyed one of us lying with him to tell his bedtime story, he was generally quite content to sleep there alone through the night. We have found that during times of stress or transition—for example, moving, a new job, or emotional strain—we usually find ourselves together in the same bed. I always feel fortunate that we have the ability to sleep together during these times. As conscientious parents we often feel that we are meeting our children's expressed needs, but what about their unexpressed ones? Part of the appeal of being close at night is the feeling that perhaps some of those are being met. I know for myself that the closeness and warmth on a cold or unsettling night is very comforting.

I think our biggest practical breakthrough was the purchase of two futons. We started with a double-size and a single. Initially, our still-nursing daughter slept between my husband and me, and our son (at age four) rolled his futon out next to ours. Some nights he "camped out" in his playroom, the mobility of the futon being ideally suited for making the gradual transition to his own space. The children, now three and five-and-a-half years, go to sleep together in their own bed and seem to be providing comfort and closeness for each other. The time seems to have returned when my husband and I will have a marital bed. It feels just as natural for us to once again have our own space as it did to bring our babies to bed with us.

The intense needs of a new baby change a mother's focus. In giving to the baby she is in turn receiving a lot of warmth and closeness. Her needs for affection may for the most part be met by her baby. Also, hormonal changes accompanying lactation (prolactin, which produces milk, inhibits estrogens) may have the effect of decreasing her sexual desire. This may all be a part of nature's plan to space children for optimal mothering. For whatever reason, babies can come between husbands and wives physically if not emotionally. There are no two ways about it, the presence of children cuts down on the ease and frequency of love-making. In addition, after putting constant energy into one's children all during the day, it may be difficult to give anymore at the end of the day. I have been fortunate that my husband believes that babies' needs come first. And yet we still have found that our need to be together to talk, to touch, cannot be put underground indefinitely. What has worked well for us from time to time is to make a "date," even if it is just setting time aside to talk alone in our own living room. The spontaneity of the "before children" relationship may temporarily be gone, but for now, a little planning goes a long way.

During trying times, we are apt to question if we are really doing what is right for our family. I then remind myself that we simply have not encountered the problems frequently associated with children's sleep. For example, our unusual sleeping arrangement has often made travelling easier. Camping in a tent was no adjustment, and when visiting relatives, we often find some little cousins joining our children in sleeping bags on the floor at the foot of our bed.

This is a bedtime story with many chapters yet to be written. For my family there will probably be revision ahead in both ideas and sleeping arrangements. Hopefully where the continuity will be is in the development of love, trust, and respect that has had its foundation in the family bed.

Suggested reading:

Touching: The Human Significance of the Skin by Ashley Montagu, Columbia University Press, New York, NY, 1971;

Magical Child by Joseph Chilton Pearce, E.P. Dutton Co., New York, NY, 1977;

The Family Bed by Tine Thevenin, P.O. Box 16004, Minneapolis, MN 55416, 1976.

An Interview with Michio Kushi

BY BARBARA JACOBS

EWJ: *I'd like to ask you about the next stage of development after weaning— that is, when a child begins to talk. Do you have any particular method that you recommend for helping a child learn to talk?*

Kushi: Children begin to learn to talk in a very natural way, making their own sounds, their own words. Let them speak in their own way, frequently. You need not teach any definite word until about three or four months. Then you gradually introduce adult words, repeating them very slowly. Children usually repeat words many times, but that is because parents talk very rapidly.

Children's brain wavelengths are different from those of adults. Children's wavelengths are much longer; when we become adults, they become shorter. So the adult's way of talking is quicker. Children's speech will be much slower, because their brain waves are longer than adults'. So, when talking to children, adults should speak more slowly, and then children can understand and will need to repeat words only one or two times, instead of many times, as children usually do.

If you speak slowly, you can still use adult words and children will understand very easily. The same idea applies to reading stories to children: Read slowly so they will understand easily. If you read slowly, after one or two times the children can memorize the story very easily.

When writing letters or numbers, use a large size so their brains, which work better with bigger sizes of objects, can comprehend better. Even with more difficult words, if larger letters are used, the children will be able to understand them easily.

The important thing to keep in mind when teaching children to speak, understand words, and read is always to consider the children's brain wavelengths and proceed slowly. Even many children who have been designated mentally retarded are actually not mentally retarded but have just been taught at the wrong tempo and with letters and numbers that are too small for them to understand completely. They have been taught at adult speed and with adult sizes of letters and objects, and therefore they cannot understand. If we use the method of proceeding slowly and using larger sizes of letters and objects, even by the age of five years the children can have a command of many adult expressions.

Of course, at the same time as this mental development takes place, children are developing physically. Physical development always precedes mental development. So the child should be active in both play and learning. The adults should not interfere in the child's physical development. For example, if parents are overprotective, or pick up a child too much who is just learning to crawl or walk, the child's physical and therefore mental development will be impaired. If a parent picks up this child for one minute, interrupting his or her crawling or walking, that means interfering with about 500 years of biological development. During the embryonic period, before birth, a baby develops at the rate of about 10 million years per day, totaling about 3 billion years of biological evolution before birth. It takes about one-and-a-half years from the time of birth until the child can stand straight, walk, and talk. This corresponds to repeating about 400 million years of human evolution. This breaks down to about 500 years per minute for the child's first one-and-a-half years from birth.

Crawling is very important to a baby, because it is through crawling that the muscles and joints are developed and strengthened. Through that kind of activity children are also developing their brains and judgment properly. When they become proficient at one stage, they can proceed normally to the next stage of physical and mental development. That is why it is very important for the child to be active and develop at his or her own pace and not be interrupted by an overprotective parent.

EWJ: *How would you explain children's widely differing speeds of development?*
Kushi: That is due to what children eat. We should not give children food that will make them mature physically too quickly. Animal food, for example, makes children mature too quickly. A diet with milk, cheese, etc., will make children grow faster physically but remain mentally undeveloped; the mental growth cannot match the physical growth. Human beings should be about one year old before standing up—even one-and-a-half years is all right. If a baby has developed teeth very early—for example, at three to five months (according to modern statistics, the average age in this country is six to seven months for first teeth to appear)—or has other signs of extremely early maturity, that is a sign of imbalance, of an excessive condition due to too high a percentage of animal protein in the diet. Animal food should be at the most only about one-eighth, or 15 percent, of the diet. Of course, you

don't need to give animal food—red meat, poultry, eggs, fish, milk, cheese—to children. They can grow very well without it.

On the other hand, some children develop very slowly. If babies aren't walking by the time they are almost two years old, that could be due to an excess of salt in their diet or not enough fresh vegetables. Too much salt makes a baby unable to expand and grow. Finally, in the case of many modern children who eat foods containing sugar, chemicals, or a large amount of fruit, the same slowness could be a sign of another kind of weakness; that is, they may be hindered mentally as well.

Parents' interference (picking the child up often, etc.) may also be a factor contributing to extremely slow development. Let's assume that the child is standing up at one year old, but that the parents have spent a total of many hours in carrying the child. That total time of "interference" (maybe months) will be added on to the child's physical development. He or she may not be walking until much later simply because his or her own normal rate of development has been tampered with. The child's mental development and ability to understand will be hindered, along with its physical growth, so it will have to catch up later mentally as well as physically. Therefore, slowness develops in three ways: too much yang (overcontractive, due to salt) food, too much yin (such as sugar, chemicals, fruit) food, too much interference by parents.

EWJ: *Earlier you mentioned the language of babies, which we consider nonsense syllables, and you emphasized that they should be allowed to play in this language freely. What is that language?*
Kushi: The language of babies is a very symbolic one. When a baby says one word, he or she is saying one word with many, many meanings. Children have many concepts but can't formulate them in precise detail. The scope of babies' concepts is actually as broad as adults', but babies' concepts are not expressed in such detail. Adult mentality makes each part of that total understanding more clear, more precise. An adult may use about ten thousand words to express the same concepts for which a child, in symbolic expression, uses only about twenty. During that period, if children are given too many fragmented adult concepts, they can't develop total understanding. So let children talk to themselves, to dogs, flowers, anything, in their own language. Then gradually the more fragmented expression of adult society will come out of that. Usually adults think that babies' minds are small, that they can't perceive as much as adults. But actually, babies' minds encompass as much as adults', even though babies don't express themselves in such a detailed way.

EWJ: *Once children have learned to talk and may have started to read, they begin school. The first requirement for that is vaccination, which many of our readers object to. What advice do you have regarding vaccination?*

Kushi: The idea behind giving immunizations is to create a sickness artificially so that the body will create a natural resistance to a second and stronger appearance of the same sickness. But why are some people more susceptible than others to the same illness? Because their daily way of life, their daily way of eating, is unhealthy. If their daily way of eating, daily way of life, is healthy, they will not get such sicknesses. There is no reason to make someone artificially sick. When this is done, there is a resistance created to that disease as a natural result, but at the same time, some other aspect of natural growth is lost. This is because the growing and developing abilities are being used for resisting, for battling that sickness. So, for that reason, we should avoid vaccinations as much as possible. The idea of using vaccinations is based on somewhat of a misconception of the natural order: Modern people think that some kind of bacteria or virus is the cause, so they plan a counterattack through artificial immunizations. But they are not actually the cause, they are only agents. The real cause is the unhealthy quality of blood, due to an unhealthy way of eating. The artificial treatment is an attempt to compensate for poor quality of blood. This represents a misconception of natural order. Many governments legally require immunizations; however, it is sometimes possible to maneuver to avoid this. France, for example, has many legal requirements for vaccinations but now in France, Belgium, and other countries there is a trend to make these vaccinations not compulsory, but available to those who want them. This civil movement is becoming more and more common, and now some countries require only smallpox vaccination, leaving the people their freedom of choice. I hope that eventually this country, too, will allow people freedom of choice [in medications]. If we are eating badly, there is definitely a need for these medications—that is natural, to become sick. If the family cannot nourish children properly by eating good food, then they may be afraid and get vaccinations. However, that vaccination may be the distant cause of future physical or mental problems. The whole point is that we should eat properly and live according to the laws of nature.

EWJ: *What do you mean when you say that our eating should be in harmony with nature?*

Kushi: That means, we eat the whole biological world. After conception, we eat the essence of the animal world—that is, mother's blood—until birth. After we are born, we continue to eat mother's blood in the form of mother's milk, which is a more diluted animal-quality food. When we stand, it means that we have reached the stage of the evolution of human beings. At that time we start to eat foods from the whole spectrum of the vegetable kingdom. By that time we have graduated from animal food eating and begin eating all vegetable-quality food, as our biological ancestors did in the evolutionary process. Grains evolved on earth at the same time as Homo sapiens. Since they constitute human beings as the human species, we include grains as the main part of our diet, and vegetables and other foods as side dishes.

EWJ: *Before we talk about school as it exists, I'd like to hear your views on the ideal school. What is the purpose of education?*

Kushi: The purpose of education (at the present time) is to make the child develop as a useful social person. But that "useful" means someone who will contribute to the progress and prosperity of society by making money, working in organizations, pursuing intellectual careers. Certainly these fields have some merit, but that is only partial progress. The primary purpose of education is to help children become healthy, happy, and strong as whole human beings, not only as social persons. For that, we need to establish their understanding of why they came here, why they were born, and what their goals are, and how to keep their health and happiness on this earth. That is understanding number one, common sense. The most important thing is to develop common sense and intuition. Second come the technical problems of how to maintain good health, how to develop judgment, how to behave, and how to deal with people. After that comes social relations. At this point some part of modern education can be helpful for the problem of what kind of technical service can be done in the future. But modern education alone is not enough. Before that kind of education, we must have a broad basic education of human beings.

At the time of grammar school all children should learn how to take care of themselves. This includes how to take care of their health and how to select and prepare their daily food. They should also know how to take care of their clothes, and know the origin of their food and clothes. They should know how to make dwellings and how to grow food; they should have an understanding of the relationships within the natural world, including that of earth to the stars. All these matters of basic common sense should be established in grammar school.

In high school this basic commonsense education should be continued, but other things are introduced, such as human relations—in the sense of learning and giving respect to elders, being loving to younger people, and dealing with people in society. High-school students should then study history, geography, social and natural sciences, and go in other intellectual directions.

Modern studies are completely fragmented. The reason for this is that there is no principle that works in all areas. From the time of grammar school through all of high school, children should be learning the universal principle. This principle is what we express as balance, or yin and yang. This principle should be a part of all aspects of their education, and it should be used in learning physics, chemistry, health problems, cooking, social science, etc. Throughout their education, that principle should always be there. Then they could finish their college-level studies by the age of seventeen or eighteen. After that they can do whatever they want to do, in social education or social experience. They can begin any kind of research work, or adventures or experiments. As far as college is concerned, that part should be using the universal principle of yin and yang in original creation. Students should write, they should discover or invent something; university education should be their own creative experience or discovery.

EWJ: *Children's growing awareness of the origin of their food and clothing, which you mentioned as a part of the grammar-school years, sounds like a basic part of any traditional culture living close to nature. What would you recommend that we, as modern Westerners, do to help our children develop a similar understanding?*
Kushi: The children's participation in the family should be a major part of early education. Let them learn basic cooking. Let them also experience sewing, and make a tour through a small factory so they can see how clothes are designed, cut, and put together. The same thing applies to carpentry and any other basic skills.

EWJ: *The school that you have been describing is really an ideal one, not having much in common with the modern academic education. How would you suggest that parents who are not totally in agreement with the public schools' way of teaching deal with the differences between the school ideology and their family life?*
Kushi: If we don't have our own school, it's fine for the children to go to public school or private school. But then home education becomes even more important. Let the children encounter any kind of chance or opportunity to learn outside of school about life and living, including making clothing, cooking, or other practical things. Parents should also be explaining to the children the order of nature, in terms of yin and yang, and letting them develop, through their own observations, a way of seeing relationships in nature and between people.

EWJ: *In many cases children are being taught one set of values at home —how to eat properly, how to behave toward others—and another, sometimes conflicting point of view in school. How can we help them to make sound* *judgments on their own?*

Kushi: First, their daily food at home should be very good. Second, children should be encouraged to understand all phenomena as expressions of balance, or yin and yang. Third, parents can, at dinnertime, simply give children a question and let them figure it out themselves. Don't tell children what not to do—such as "You shouldn't eat school lunches" or "You should not learn that." Let the children select for themselves and experience what they want. But when they have some experience, there is a result. When that result comes (for example, if children eat some ice cream or candy and later don't feel so well), ask them, "Why do you feel bad today? What do you think is the cause? Did you eat some ice cream or candy?" Then the children will understand.

EWJ: *Modern education seems to emphasize competitiveness. I remember how important grades were. How do you see the natural differences in people, the personal abilities that are sometimes overlooked in a school situation or even at home?*

Kushi: Even genetic factors, such as DNA, are constantly changing. Nothing stays the same, nothing is identical. Even in the case of twins of the same sex, the space occupied in the mother's womb is different, the time of delivery is different. Each fetus in the womb selects different qualities of food from the mother's blood. Plus the mother's daily eating is different. Seasons and activity are different. So all people are different. No one is superior in all ways to other people.

When the children are evaluated, it is done with a narrow scope. Some children have an excellent school record, but that is only one small part of the whole person. The standard of present-day evaluations is very conceptual and one-sided. If children have a good mechanical memory, then they will be high scorers. But this kind of memory is only a very small part. More important are children's insights, their broad understanding and clear judgment. Those things do not appear on school records. Even more important is their physical, mental, and spiritual health. That, again, doesn't appear on school records.

Children need guidance and encouragement from their parents. The parents should encourage the children to do whatever they like to do in the future. "Do your best in school, in society , in whatever you like to do, and don't worry about competition. When you do your best in what you really want to do, that is the best." Some children go to school and get a D, others may get an A. The most important thing is who was putting forth their best effort. The child's ability is most important, and the marks received are only of secondary importance.

Many great world leaders had very bad school records. Parents should give guidance in these matters, because the school doesn't make provisions for it. So you can totally erase any idea of competition. Just encourage children to do their best, whether in school or in their responsibilities at home. When they put forth their best effort, it doesn't matter whether their marks in school are the best or the worst—they have done wonderfully.

Observing Your Child's Development

BY BARBARA JACOBS

T he following article is based on notes taken at a lecture delivered by Michio Kushi to a group of young Boston mothers.

Diagnosis

In watching over your child's development along the lines of his or her own innate abilities, it is helpful to recognise his or her constitutional tendencies. A very yang, powerfully built child with the potential to become an explorer should not be forced to prepare for the career of a fine artist, which a more yin, highly sensitive child would take to spontaneously—and vice versa. Children's external features offer some clues to the internal forces that will later blossom in their choice of self-expression as adults. Obviously, each tendency has its advantages and disadvantages. I wish to emphasize that the question of yin and yang tendencies is not a matter of "good" or "bad," "right" or "wrong," or any other judgmental concept. These natural tendencies need to be nurtured and balanced within the variety of a universe that is composed of unique individuals, all of them contributing to the harmonious and dynamic balance of society.

Extremes of yin and yang, however, can cause problems for an individual in relating to others and maintaining a balanced state of health. The following clues—starting from the top of the head, moving down the face, then out to the hands—indicate tendencies that mothers should be aware of when choosing their children's food.

The first thing we can notice is the general shape of the child's head. Newborns' heads are often slightly lopsided—larger on one side than the other. After the age of one month, however, the shape normally becomes more symmetrical. An infant with the left (yin) side of the head expanded will develop an affinity for artistic or intellectual pursuits. If the right (yang) side of the head is larger, the child will tend to become a more physical or practical type of person.

In certain cases, the back (yang) of the child's head is relatively large, indicating a yang condition. If such children eat a diet including an undue proportion of animal food, such as eggs and meat, they may become very quarrelsome and even violent. In such cases try reducing the amount of animal food you give them—always being careful, of course, to provide them with a balanced diet that includes the essential nutrients for growth (such as protein and calcium) through a proper combination of whole grains, beans, and fresh vegetables.

Conversely, an infant whose head is expanded in the front (yin) may become sluggish or depressed if given excessive amounts of more yin foods, such as fruit and milk products. By watching the behavioral effects of changing your child's diet, you can observe his or her peaceful and healthy growth.

The amount of hair on the head at birth also indicates yin and yang constitutional tendencies, which are a manifestation of the mother's food intake while pregnant. Of course, the hereditary tendencies of the embryo—determined by the chemistry of the father's sperm cell and the mother's ovum—affect what kinds of nourishment the growing embryo will absorb or reject from its mother's bloodstream. However, these factors are less easy to control than the mother's choice of food. The growing embryo is constituted primarily of the nutrients it absorbs from the mother's bloodstream, and they in turn are a product of what type of food the mother ingests. Thus, mothers who typically consume substantial quantities of yin (such as tropical fruit or fruit juices, vitamin pills, and other medications) will give birth to infants with long (yin) hair. Babies whose mothers have eaten a more centered diet, based on the traditional staple of cereal grains, do not have much hair on their heads when they are born.

The hair on the head grows in a spiral pattern centering on a point toward the back of the skull. If this point is located on the left (yin) side, the individual tends toward more aesthetic or philosophical kinds of pursuits. Giving such infants large quantities of yin foods may exaggerate their innate tendencies to an extreme of dreaminess and reluctance to participate in physical activities. Infants whose hair spirals lie to the right will be more active and outgoing. If given too much yang food, they may exhibit aggressive and very thoughtless behavior. If you reduce their intake of salt and animal food, you may be pleasantly surprised.

Many children are now being born with two or more spirals. This phenomenon can be traced to the pregnant mothers' adherence to the predominant modern dietary pattern, which includes extremes of yin and yang in large amounts, ranging from heavy consumption of meat to highly chemicalized products and medication. As they mature, infants with more than one hair spiral will evince difficulty in focusing on a direction in life; often they will vacillate between suddenly shifting moods of passivity and aggression. You can greatly help such people by making available to them a diet of more centered foods, emphasizing the traditional staple of cereals—in the form of whole grain bread, rice, buckwheat, cornmeal, etc.

The uppermost facial characteristic indicative of yin or yang is the shape of the eyebrows. Eyebrows sloping up toward the temples are more yang; eyebrows that slope downward are more yin.

Relatively large (yin) eyes are associated with artistic sensibilities; smaller eyes indicate strength of will. Another obvious indication of a person's relatively yin or yang internal condition is the location of the pupil of the eye. Most infants are born with their pupils located near the lower (yang) eyelid, rather than centered between the two eyelids. This reflects the fact that children are more yang (active, small, alert) than adults. If the pupil is located nearer to the upper (yin) eyelid, this means that the individual is suffering from an extremely yin condition: the eyeball has shifted upward because of pressure caused by overexpansion of body tissues and fluids. In such cases intake of liquids, sugars, and other yin foods that metabolize into water should be kept to a minimum until the condition improves.

The lips are the beginning of the digestive tract. Expanded lips indicate a weakened digestive system that has been dilated by excessive consumption of yin foods. Very careful attention to a balanced and moderate diet is to be recommended in such instances. The digestive system, situated in the soft, front (yin) part of the body, largely reflects the contribution to the embryo's development from the mother's (yin) egg cell. Thus, tendencies toward intestinal difficulties (such as duodenal ulcers and Krohn's disease) often run in a matrilineal pattern. The nervous system—centralized in the spine, which runs up the back (yang) side of the body—is more influenced by the contribution of the father's (yang) sperm cell to the embryo. To create and maintain a sound nervous system, adequate minerals in the diet and physical activity are essential.

The firmness of the baby's grip is a clear gauge of the strength of the circulatory system, which develops between the digestive and nervous systems. Long fingers are associated with aesthetic talents, and shorter fingers are a sign of strong, practical types.

Education

There is no justification for scolding or hitting a child. When children are "bad," it is you who think so. Children themselves have no concept of "bad," "wrong," "evil," and so forth. Such illusory ideas are only manifestations of the peculiar mental illness that adults term "civilization." In reality, when you hit your child for being "bad," you are actually angry at yourself for not being a better parent.

Sloppy children are the product of careless parents or of their opposites—over solicitous parents. Pampered, spoiled children never learn how to take care of themselves. Give your children the opportunity to learn the basic habits of neatness by picking up after themselves and generally taking care of their things.

Allow your children to help you cook, clean house, or watch over younger brothers and sisters. These tasks need never be imposed as if they were duties or responsibilities. Rather than being too serious about life's normal activities, teach them to participate in your work in the spirit of play. Children who are forced to do things will inevitably rebel and start concealing their spontaneity. When you force children to lie to you this way, you create a communication gap that may grow into a serious separation between generations. Try to adapt a more relaxed and happy approach.

Almost every family in the modern world watches television. In my opinion, reliance on television as a mechanical babysitter or time killer is not a wise practice, because dependence on television affects the child's natural powers of imagination adversely and tends to foster laziness. You might try turning the time when your children watch television to their advantage, by answering the questions they will naturally have about what they see. From time to time, ask them what they think of the advertisements, the situations portrayed, the people's behavior, and so forth.

But I suggest that, rather than watching a lot of television, you read to your children regularly. Also, allow them to make up stories of their own and then to draw them or write them down. And give them a chance to read to you, often. Reading aloud was a very common practice in the past, when families were less passive about their education. The activity of reading aloud, which is comparable to singing or chanting, is beneficial to health.

Of course, there is no reason to constantly participate in your children's activities. They are entitled to their privacy, just like adults. Where the child's and adult's world intermesh, however, you have an opportunity to show them, through example, ways of polite acknowledgment. Children enjoy learning the basics of politeness, such as saying "Good morning," "How are you?" "Thank you very much." If you show them how to express some form of thanks before and after meals, you will be giving them the foundation for an attitude of appreciation towards all of life.

Point out the colors of flowers and other beauties of nature. Encourage their curiosity by asking them questions (for example, why something is shaped the way it is). When you go out shopping, take your children along sometimes and explain what you are doing. Ask them what they think about the way people act. If you stimulate their natural development this way, you will see them grow into adults who will give happiness to many people.

Whatever your children want to do, encourage them to try their hardest. Although anyone can learn to do a given activity with a modicum of skill, don't coerce children to go against their natural inclinations and tendencies. Whatever you do never discourage a child's dream.

Natural Childcare

Natural Health Insurance
What Determines Your Child's Health

BY BARBARA AND LEONARD JACOBS

Whippen raising a child using a natural or macrobiotic approach it is necessary to anticipate the child's possible sicknesses before they arise. You need to understand which factors contribute to health and which ones may create an imbalance resulting in sickness. It is also necessary to observe the child's expression, color, and other facial signs to be able to understand his or her current condition and see developing problems. For instance, if the child's facial color becomes pale—indicating blood and respiratory congestion—you can expect some physical symptoms to develop like tiredness, irritability, a cold, indigestion, or diarrhea. If the child constantly has a runny nose, you can be sure that he or she is overeating and probably taking too much bread, cookies, and juice. The runny nose indicates potential problems with the digestive system and possibly a mineral imbalance. In other words, the systems are completely interrelated and the parents have to be able to anticipate minor symptoms rather than waiting for crises.

The first and major influence on the course of the child's health is the mother's health and diet prior to and during pregnancy. Of course, the father's health and quality of sperm are also very important, but it is the mother who during pregnancy creates the child's basic constitutional strength. The first three months of pregnancy are especially important, and the mother must both satisfy her cravings as well as eat a sensible and nutritious diet. During the beginning of pregnancy it's very common to think too much about what you should eat. Many women follow nutritional guidelines that are set up for an average person, not tailored to their own unique conditions. Many cravings—for salty, sweet, sour, or animal foods—will arise during the first two to three months of pregnancy due to the rapid growth of the embryo from a single cell to a small organism. A wide variety of nutrients is necessary for this growth, and the mother's blood has to contain all of them.

It's generally advisable to satisfy these intuitive cravings but instead of relying on foods such as meat, sugar, ice cream, or soda, they should be satisfied with less harmful and more nourishing types of food. For instance, if you crave animal food such as meat or chicken, you may need more protein. You can try fish, seitan, tofu, tempeh, or beans. If you crave pickles and ice cream, this may be because of a need for more calcium (sour foods help to mobilize your body's own stores of calcium), and you can try sauerkraut or other good-quality pickles along with sesame seeds, tahini, turnip greens, sea vegetables, or other foods rich in calcium. In any case, along with finding nutritious foods which satisfy these extreme taste cravings, it's best to eat at least 30 percent whole grains, a small amount of miso soup, some cooked vegetables, and salad every day throughout your pregnancy. Most women find that after the third or fourth month they can return to their usual diet of 50 to 60 percent whole grains and other foods including cooked vegetables, beans, sea vegetables, seeds, fruits, and a small amount of fish. Beverages during pregnancy can include barley and bancha teas as well as small amounts of herb teas or fruit juices depending on your own personal taste. It's best not to take any alcohol, caffeine, honey, and sugared beverages during your pregnancy.

Besides diet, a calm environment is a very important factor in a healthy and comfortable pregnancy. Try to avoid violent movies, loud or chaotic music, and stressful situations. It is also a good idea to maintain some type of yoga or other exercise regimen, such as walking or bicycling. Your health during pregnancy is your child's best insurance for future health and actually is the best immunization against future sicknesses.

The birth experience itself is the next opportunity to foster your child's strength and vitality. Whether your child is born at home or in the hospital it is best to avoid any kind of drug or medication. A sitting or squatting position (as was the general practice until comparatively recently) allows for an easier delivery with the least strain on the mother and baby. Once the child is delivered it's best not to cut the umbilical cord until after it has stopped pulsating and the child has begun to breathe on its own. Also, it's best not to wash off the vernix or use silver nitrate in the eyes. You can pat the child with a diaper or thin towel, wrap him or her in a blanket, and leave the child to rest next to the mother.

Hospitals usually administer what is called the Apgar test to judge the child's health. This tests foot reflexes and otherwise determines that the baby has a normal human constitution. In addition to this type of examination there are several other points to consider. Has the child cried at least enough to discharge any mucus from the throat and nose? If not you will have to use an infant suction cup to remove any mucus. Also, the whites of the eyes should be clear and slightly steely blue in color. If the infant's eyes are open you can also check that the iris is not totally in the center of the eye but that some of the white shows above the iris. These signs indicate a healthy and vital nervous system regardless of other tests of the child's reflexes. Next check how many spirals the child has on the top of the head. Metaphorically and possibly even literally, the spiral reflects the actual physical constitution of the child. If there is more than one spiral this indicates that there was difficulty during the mother's pregnancy—some trauma or radical change in diet or lifestyle during the previous nine months. A child with more than one spiral may have a tendency towards some future difficulties or illnesses, but if watched closely he or she may develop strong leadership or artistic qualities later in life. If there is only one spiral, observe how tight it is and whether it's toward the right or left, toward the top or more towards the bottom of the head. (Of course, the head may be slightly misshapen depending on the length of time the baby was in the birth canal, and it may take up to six months before the position of the spiral is really permanent.) If the spiral is more toward the right or lower down on the head, the child will be generally more active and outgoing. If towards the left or higher up on the head, he or she may be more artistic or intellectual; this type of child, being more sensitive, will require more moderation in his or her diet. If the spiral is in the center the child will be more balanced in outlook and activities.

Next look at your child's ears. If the lower part of the lobe is detached from the side of the head and the ear lays flat (against the head), this means the child has great natural stamina and resistance against sickness or other difficulties. If the ears stick out (as a result of the mother eating too many raw fruits, citrus fruits, or raw vegetables), this child may have more tendencies toward skin problems, allergies, and other childhood sicknesses. If there is no lower lobe or if it is attached (because the mother ate too much animal food or not enough mineral-rich vegetables), the child may be prone to fevers and have a tendency to self-preoccupation.

The next area to examine on the newborn infant is the palm. The three major lines that indicate the conditions of the heart and circulatory system, and the nervous and digestive systems will be clear, long, and deep if the child has strength in all these systems.

Even though all these areas point to the child's overall constitutional strength, to some extent the mother can still create greater vitality in her baby through her diet while nursing.

Another observation to make about your child is the way he or she sleeps. If the child sleeps on his or her stomach, there may be a problem with digestion, or a tendency toward digestive problems. The mother, while she is nursing her baby, can change this condition. If the baby sleeps on his or her back, with the arms up over the head, this is a sign of a healthy constitution—openness and peacefulness. This is like a flower growing and is an indication that the child will be relatively free of sicknesses.

If after examining your child you feel that he or she is generally healthy and has a strong, sound constitution, you should have very few problems and no need for a doctor's care or for immunizations. This does not mean, however, that the child will never become sick. Young children, because they are so active and are growing so quickly, are constantly adjusting and discharging any imbalance, whether from embryological imbalances (from the mother's diet), from the mother's diet while nursing, or from their own diet after they are weaned. These simple discharges are generally not serious but instead are signs of the child's natural strength. For instance, if the mother begins eating many desserts or fruit the quality of her milk will change. The baby may then get a runny nose or diaper rash. The simplest way to correct this is through the mother's diet, not necessarily by using any external treatments on the baby. Some of the symptoms the baby may have in the first year are fevers, skin problems, colic, or colds. These discharge/adjustment-type symptoms are usually caused by extremes of two types: either too much salt, animal food, baked or overly cooked food, or overactivity of the mother (yang), or on the other hand, sugar, fruits, raw vegetables, or too much liquid in the mother's diet (yin). Excess of yang will produce redness, high fevers, dry coughs, irritability, constant hunger, and in some cases inability to sleep for more than two or three hours at a time. Excesses of yin will bring about low but persistent fevers, a runny nose, skin problems, weak crying or whining, weak appetite, and irritability.

If the mother makes adjustments in her diet, usually the baby's condition will immediately correct itself. With diaper rash, especially if the skin gets very raw and sore, arrowroot powder, calendula powder, or cream will soothe the skin. If the child has a minor fever, that is, of 103 degrees F. or less, it is usually sufficient for the mother to change her diet in order to correct the problem. (You can easily take an infant's temperature by putting the thermometer under the armpit, keeping it there for four to five minutes, and adding 1 degree F. to the temperature shown.) If the temperature is over 103 degrees F. it is important to use more specific methods to reduce the fever as quickly as possible—in fact, at this time it is advisable to take the child's temperature every three to four hours to be sure the condition doesn't get out of control. A fever of 104 degrees F. or 105 degrees F. for more than twelve hours could result in problems including very serious illnesses such as spinal meningitis.

Although a high fever like this is often a result of yang excesses it may have been caused by excess yin such as some drugs administered at birth or some medication taken during the pregnancy or even before conception. A high fever is in fact the body's natural attempt to discharge (burn off) some strong excess. Be sure that during the fever the child takes plenty of liquid or nurses more often to prevent dehydration. Also, the mother can try drinking some slightly more sweet foods such as rice malt, beer, or warmed fruit juices. If possible give the child some amesake drink, sweetened bancha tea, or the cooked juice of grated daikon radish. Fresh tofu or a chlorophyl plaster can also be applied behind the child's ears. A tofu plaster is squeezed tofu mixed with about 15 to 20 percent white flour and a small amount of grated fresh ginger. A chlorophyl plaster is made by mashing fresh greens in a suribachi.

While watching the fever you will notice that it generally goes up at night and down during the day. You will know that the fever has broken if it doesn't go up at night or in fact begins to go down. In extreme cases, with a persistent fever, you may have to wrap the child in a wet sheet, sponge him or her off with a cool wet washcloth, or even put the child in a lukewarm tub. However, if the child loses his or her appetite and the fever does not break after twelve hours, seek professional help such as a holistically-oriented pediatrician. It may be a good idea to make friends with some medical professional—someone you trust to whom you can go for reassurance or specific treatments when you are unable to figure out for yourself what is best to do. Although your child may develop various types of minor sicknesses, with proper diet and an understanding of diagnosis it's certainly possible to avoid serious complications or the types of problems most of us experienced when we were children.

Eating Well, the Best Vaccine

BY LEONARD JACOBS

Q: *What is your opinion of the value of vaccinations/immunizations for childhood diseases? I have been eating a natural foods diet for the past two years but don't want to take any chances with my daughter's well-being.*

—S. Catallano
Allentown, Pennsylvania

A: In order to make an intelligent decision on the pros and cons of immunizations, we first have to understand the meaning of sickness and disease; then we can prevent or cure any sickness through the balanced application of yin and yang. This understanding will also help us see what role immunization can play in the well-being of our children. However, I want to emphasize that the following ideas are presented merely as my opinions based on seven years of study, observation, and treatment of my own children. Your personal decision on whether to immunize your child must be your own.

Sickness results from an imbalance between a person's inner environment and the external world, which is manifested in symptoms ranging from unhappiness, depression, or fear, to fevers, aches and pains, or malfunctioning organs. In general, sicknesses fall into two categories: eliminating (or balancing) sicknesses, in which the body automatically rids itself of excesses (e.g., colds, fevers, skin eruptions, diarrhea, anger) and degenerative (or chronic) diseases, in which the body is so weakened from a long period of abuse that it can no longer discharge the accumulated excesses and begins to degenerate (arthritis, diabetes, heart disease, colitis, cancer, schizophrenia). These two categories of sickness also apply to childhood diseases. It is possible to prevent these diseases if we understand their causes. Vaccinations for creating an artificial immunity against sickness then become unnecessary; we can avoid the problem entirely by establishing and maintaining a healthy balance between the child and his or her environment.

Vaccinations are routinely given for the following supposedly "infectious" diseases: tetanus, diphtheria, pertussis (whooping cough), polio, measles, mumps, smallpox, and rubella (German measles). All these diseases are supposed to be caused by germs, that is, bacteria or viruses, which are thought of as external agents that invade the body.

In the 1860s Louis Pasteur developed the germ theory of disease which, in brief, claims that microscopic organisms of a pathogenic nature can invade a human organism and cause disease. This theory met with mixed reactions in the medical community when it was first introduced; but because of the extremely analytical and mechanistic intellectual climate at that time in Europe and America on the brink of the Industrial Age, it was eventually accepted and has been further refined up until the present.

From the most primitive life forms, viruses and bacteria, to the most evolved cells of the cerebrum, our bodies are composed of a constantly evolving continuum of life forms. The primitive life forms are not our enemies, but rather constitute the evolutionary origin of our body cells and the eventual future of our bodies as they return to the soil after death. Pasteur was aware that even fermentation (which he studied extensively while formulating his germ theory) only occurs in injured, bruised, or dead material, and that bacteria are a natural result of fermentation, not the cause. Nevertheless, modern medicine sees infectious disease caused by an external substance attacking an "innocent" host organism. I would suggest, rather, that an internally weakened host organism, trying to deal with constant discharge sicknesses, begins to degenerate and eventually produces harmful bacteria and viruses (germs), which are then observed by science and diagnosed as being the cause of the sickness.

"Dr. Antoine Bechamp observed that germs evolve out of decaying cells they helped to build, and take part in the decomposing of the ever-changing life substance and help to form it into material usable again by nature. Thus when germs are found within a sick body, it is not that they entered from outside and caused the disease. It is because they developed from the decaying cells within the body and have an important part to play in helping to handle the toxins taken into the body from without" (*Don't Get Stuck* by Hannah Allen, Healthways Publications, Pearsall, Texas, p. 20). The so-called infectious diseases are actually discharge sicknesses which can be prevented by maintaining a healthy organism through normal exercise and a balanced diet with a minimum of processed or chemicalized foods. Then, even when your child is in the presence of a so-called epidemic of some "infectious" disease, he or she will have complete immunity. Immunity is completely *natural* and not a rare privilege to be bought with money or acquired from the technological arsenal.

In addition to this alternate theory concerning germs and immunity, there are several other points concerning immunization which you should consider before deciding on whether to give your child vaccinations. As sanitary conditions improved throughout the world, the incidence of "infectious" diseases declined at a very rapid rate. Vaccinations were introduced at a time when water and food supplies were being handled in much more hygienic ways, and vaccinations were most likely more incidental than causal in the reduction of the prevalence of childhood and other "infectious" diseases. In fact, according to the *World Health Statistics Annual*, 1973-1976, volume 2 (published by the World Health Organization, Geneva, Switzerland), there has been a steady decline of infectious diseases in most "developing" countries regardless of the percentage of immunizations administered in these countries. It appears that generally improved conditions of sanitation are largely responsible for preventing "infectious" diseases.

Another basic factor involved in immunity (the natural ability to maintain balance with the environment) is whether the child is nursed on mother's milk or cow's milk. During the first two or three days of nursing, before the actual milk is produced, the mother produces a clear, milk-like substance called colostrum. This substance contains many of the antibodies and other substances necessary to induce natural immunity in the infant. If the child is bottlefed on cow's milk, however, this colostrum is never consumed. Furthermore, the consumption of cow's milk often causes allergic reactions in children, which represent the beginning of the discharge sicknesses that eventually culminate in bacterial and "infectious" diseases.

Our education instills an almost superstitious belief in the current tenets of science; however, it is possible to think for oneself and consider alternate theories in the light of one's own experience. Sickness and disease can be perceived quite differently from the orthodox theories of modern medicine. The germ theory of disease may be incorrect, and other factors may be responsible for the relative increases or decreases of childhood diseases. But in case you are still convinced of the effectiveness of immunizations and feel that, in order to play it safe, you should give your child certain vaccinations, I will offer a little more detail on vaccine serums.

"Active immunization is based on the theory that the injection of an antigen (disease product) into the body will stimulate antibody formation against the disease. These antibodies will then work to fight off pathogenic bacteria in the future, just as they do in a person who has previously had the disease. The immunizing substance is prepared from either a live weakened strain of the disease agent, or from processed, inactivated components of the agent" (*Immunizations: Are They Necessary?*, by Randy Neustaedter, Hering Family Health Clinic,

Berkeley, California). That sounds safe enough, but have you considered the origin of these antigens? Remember how the famous swine flu vaccine was produced from rotten, infected eggs? The other antigens are obtained from similar sources, although information regarding the origins of the most common children's vaccines is not generally publicized. I did discover, however, from the British National Anti-Vaccination League, the following information: "Materials from which vaccines and serums are produced: (1) rotten horse blood, for diphtheria toxin and antitoxin; (2) pulverized felt hats, for tetanus serum; (3) sweepings from vacuum cleaners, for asthma and hay fever serums; (4) pus from sores on diseased cows for smallpox serums; (5) mucus from the throats of children with colds and whooping cough, for whooping cough serum; (6) decomposed fecal matter from typhoid patients, for typhoid serum." The Salk polio vaccine is derived from the infected brains of monkeys.

No wonder that a major reason for avoiding immunizations has been that these injections have often caused serious sickness and occasionally death. Deaths from smallpox inoculations are more widespread on an annual basis than actual cases of smallpox in the world. Polio has occurred following diphtheria and pertussis immunizations as well as after the administrations of the polio vaccine itself.

Artificially introducing diseased substances into a child's body can result in extreme reactions; often, general resistance is lowered for years following immunizations, and occasionally chronic disease can be traced back to an initial dose of a vaccine or serum.

Another point to consider in evaluating the truthfulness of immunization campaigns is the economic motive of the pediatricians and pharmaceutical companies. Drug companies have a definite vested interest in the administration of inoculations and often work closely with doctors and clinics on "educational" programs as well as giving kick-back subsidies to the medical establishment. At the same time, newspapers and other media that regularly depend on pharmaceutical advertising tend to suppress or ignore any negative developments concerning adverse reactions to immunization programs. (Very little information was published in the daily newspapers about the increasing prevalence of polio following the Salk polio vaccine program begun in the middle 1950s.) Iatrogenic (doctor-induced) diseases on a clinical level are rarely reported on in general yet are responsible for between 40 and 60 percent of all disease complications in hospitals or clinics. Many of these iatrogenic diseases are caused by pharmaceutical products, specifically vaccination immunizations.

Discharge sicknesses—and eventually degenerative diseases—are often caused by the continual injection of booster shots of vaccinations. Since many doctors do not understand the mechanism of sickness and immunity, they continue to rely on the dualistic (and therefore destructive) germ theory of disease that only serves to perpetuate the incidence of childhood diseases.

Natural immunity includes the ability to accommodate most discharge sicknesses. But, as mentioned earlier, a long series of these acute sicknesses may eventually produce chronic degenerative diseases. If there is a problem of constantly recurring illnesses, one should stop and ask what factors in the child's diet or mode of living are producing the constant imbalances that underlie his or her sicknesses.

Childhood Illnesses

BY LEONARD JACOBS

Q: *How are "childhood illnesses" different from adult sicknesses?
What should I do about the sicknesses for which my pediatrician tells me
I have to give my child vaccinations?*

—S. Starke
Albuquerque, New Mexico

A: Basically, there are three causes of childhood illnesses: (1) the growing child is discharging the residue of an embryological imbalance; (2) there is a temporary imbalance in the child's daily diet or environment; (3) a chronically imbalanced diet or lifestyle has resulted in degeneration of the tissue, organs, or nervous system. Contrary to popular belief, germs are not the cause of "infectious" childhood diseases; rather, germs arise in an already degenerating organism that is trying to discharge toxins.

In *Pasteur: Plagiarist, Imposter* (Natural Hygiene Society, 1942), R. B. Pearson states that "Bacteria found in man and animals do not cause disease—they have the same function as those found in the soil, or in sewage, or elsewhere in nature; they are there to rebuild dead or diseased tissues, or rework body wastes, and it is well known that they will not (or cannot) attack healthy tissue." At a conference in 1979 at Tufts University, Alec Burton, O.D., said, "No one will deny the existence of germs and other microorganisms, or that they are intimately associated with certain diseases. They may be secondary or tertiary factors, but they are not the primary and fundamental causes of diseases. They are intimately associated with, and necessary to, the evolution of some diseases, but *the condition of the host is the primary factor*. Bacteria are so important to life that we cannot survive without them. They take on certain characteristics, depending on the environment in which they find themselves. Germs don't cause disease— disease creates an environment favorable to the proliferation of germs."

It seems quite likely, therefore, that childhood sicknesses are the result of factors other than invading pathogenic microorganisms. In order to discuss some of these other factors I will first give an historical sketch of the incidence of childhood diseases, and then talk about some of the mechanisms of immunity. Finally, I will consider how childhood diseases differ from those of adults.

An article on "Infectious Diseases in Primitive Societies" in *Science* February 14, 1975, states that many modern diseases do not occur in the few primitive societies that are still uncontaminated by technological civilization. Also, many types of infectious diseases have appeared in history only recently. Smallpox did not exist before 100 A.D., measles before 600 A.D.; there was no cholera before 1500 A.D., and no widespread incidence of polio before 1887. Lifestyles and food patterns (such as the introduction of citrus fruits to Europe after the Crusades and the steady rise in sugar consumption after the discovery of the West Indies) have been changing in an increasingly unnatural direction since the eleventh century. These facts (see *Diseases in Antiquity* by Don Brothwell and A.T. Sandison) suggest that modern society, with its artificial environment and diet, may be the significant factor in the cause of modern sicknesses.

The dramatic increase in children's diseases began in the middle 1800s and continued until the 1920s. Whether the drastic reduction of these diseases after 1920 was caused by improved sanitary procedures or by medical discoveries is a disputed point. In *Medical Nemesis* Ivan Illich marshals evidence for the former view, that sanitation was in fact responsible for the recent decline in the incidence of childhood diseases, for which modern medicine claims credit.

Even if immunizations can effectively counteract these sicknesses in some cases, there may very well be more natural and less dangerous ways to prevent your child from getting them. First among these, of course, is proper diet.

Unfortunately, as evidenced by the recent swine flu immunization program, it is very difficult to avoid pressure exerted by "experts" within the medical establishment. By playing upon parents' fears, doctors make it very difficult for them to choose not to immunize their children.

Some information doctors seldom give parents is that many of these diseases are extremely rare. The incidence of diphtheria in North America is one case per million people; for tetanus, one case per 600,000 (and 73 percent of those cases occur in people over the age of fifty); in 1974 there were seven cases of polio in the entire United States. Mumps, chicken pox, measles and German measles are much more common—about 50 percent of all American children have had these illnesses by the time they reach fifteen—but the symptoms are not very serious and complications are quite rare.

Recently, the incidence of measles has been increasing again among school-age children, and the U.S. Department of Health, Education, and Welfare, along with the Federal Center for Disease Control, is involved in an all-out effort to immunize 20 million American children (90 percent of all school children) against "seven infectious childhood diseases" (polio, measles, diphtheria, tetanus, whooping cough, German measles, mumps). It is highly likely that this massive immunization program will produce many serious side-effects, as happened with the swine flu fiasco. There are no statistical studies correlating the incidence of serious side-effects with routine immunizations, but it is known that side-effects, mimicking the disease itself, do occur quite often. The swine flu program demonstrated the potential dangers of a national immunization program.

Another example of the danger of immunization is the polio (Salk vaccine) program of twenty years ago. The article "Lessons of the Swine Flu Debacle" in *The Nation* (February 12, 1977) had this to say: "In April 1955, hundreds of children who were given the dangerous Salk vaccine contracted the disease, and many of them died. The investigative report was delivered to HEW in June. The secretary of HEW resigned in July and the director of the National Institutes of Health shortly thereafter. The Surgeon General of the Public Health Service elected early retirement to the drug industry employment the following year." In his book *Margin of Safety* John Rowan Wilson, (Doubleday, 1963), documents the tragic consequences of the Salk vaccine. He attributes the polio disaster to a mixture of scientific arrogance, political maneuvering, limited professional capability, and excessive public awe of the scientific establishment.

The decisions reached by research scientists, doctors, and pediatricians are clearly influenced by factors such as self-interest or economic ties to the pharmaceutical companies. According to *The New York Times* (June 28, 1976), the drug industry spends over $1 billion per year in advertising and promotion for their pharmaceuticals. Any evaluation of the advisability of immunization against childhood diseases must take this fact into account.

Scientists do agree that pathogenic microorganisms cannot live in a healthy body. One way the body develops immunity is through a wide variety of antibodies produced by the thymus, a gland of the endocrine-hormonal system which becomes inactive after puberty.

Thus it is important for a maturing child to be exposed to a wide variety of stimuli and possible "germs" in order to elicit the production of antibodies which will give lasting immunity to sickness. The temporary symptoms of "childhood illnesses" can be seen as a natural result of the thymic production of antibodies; by the time the thymus has ceased to function, "childhood illnesses" no longer appear.

Another reason children have their own category of sicknesses is that growing children quickly discharge any excess they have consumed. This natural process of discharge produces symptoms such as fever, coughing, swelling, rashes, and so forth. In fact, these symptoms are usually related to the lymph system, through which the thymus circulates antibodies. Unfortunately, removal of children's tonsils (part of the lymph system's filtering mechanism), which was encouraged by medical experts, impairs the natural regulation of the lymph system; this fashionable operation is often the first step toward creating susceptibility to allergies, infectious diseases, and general health problems. There is a well-documented relationship between the likelihood of contracting polio and a history of tonsillectomy. It is possible that this operation, which usually follows the child having been raised on cow's milk (rather than mother's milk), is largely responsible for the more acute symptoms of childhood illnesses and the serious complications that sometimes result from these sicknesses. In my opinion, excessive consumption of dairy food (cow's milk) by today's children is a major factor in the development of symptoms associated with difficulty in discharging excess mucus. Tonsillectomy suppresses those symptoms and impairs the body's mechanism for discharging toxins thus seriously damaging our ability to heal ourselves.

The Immunization Debate

BY LEONARD JACOBS

One of the first decisions a parent has to face is whether or not to immunize or vaccinate a child. For those of us involved with natural foods and a natural lifestyle, however, it has been very difficult to obtain useful information on how to deal with this problem.

The M.D.'s, of course, are unwilling to consider any alternative to immunization—on the contrary, they overwhelmingly support vaccinations—while schools, public health officials, and teachers all follow and reinforce the doctors' opinion. Parents who seek an alternative are completely on their own. Although many of us would not hesitate to ignore current medical advice in matters affecting our own health, we are not quite as willing to trust our judgment or intuition when it comes to making decisions that concern the well-being of our children. My own experience as a parent has taught me that immunizations are not essential, but this does not mean that a child who has not been immunized will not get sick. Before we decide not to immunize our children, we must understand very clearly what is involved.

When we choose to vaccinate a child, what we have done is to give a doctor, a pharmaceutical company, and a research scientist the responsibility for our child's health; we have refused to take the full responsibility ourselves. Modern medicine continually tries to convince us to hand over our responsibilities to a professional. It tells us that we are not qualified to make important decisions ourselves. Yet, over the years, I have found that these professionals are not nearly as necessary as they might want us to believe.

Many people have asked me, "Should I or shouldn't I vaccinate my child?" Obviously, I can't give a flat yes or no. The really important question here concerns responsibility. If you decide not to vaccinate your children and they then develop measles, mumps, chicken pox, polio or whatever, are you prepared to deal with these diseases with a total approach to the problem and can you cure the particular symptoms involved? Of course I'm not saying that your children will develop these sicknesses if you don't vaccinate them, but the decision not to vaccinate carries with it a responsibility to bear any possible consequences. I get the impression that many people have an ostrich attitude towards the whole question, and somehow assume that merely by deciding not to go along with the medical establishment they have somehow waved a magic wand that will keep all future health problems at bay. Their attitude is just as irresponsible as that of the M.D.s who support vaccination but ignore their responsibility for the aftereffects. There are many drawbacks to immunization, which I will tell you about, but before I mention them I want you to realize how important this question of responsibility is.

In the middle of the nineteenth century, the scientific community became very concerned with germs, viruses, and bacteria. Around 1860, Louis Pasteur, who developed pasteurization and sterilization, did much of the early work on the germ theory of disease. Many of our modern ideas concerning infectious and contagious disease are founded on Pasteur's work.

Pasteur's discoveries were actually nothing new. Many of his experimental techniques had been duplicated in traditional kitchens for hundreds of years. Koji, miso, yogurt, and other fermented foods are all made with the help of "contaminating bacteria," by the same bacterial process that serves as the basis of Pasteur's germ theory of disease. However, the growth of bacteria in a living environment is much different from the growth of bacteria that have been isolated in sterile petri dishes for laboratory study.

Bacteria are all around us. Your homes are filled with bacteria: Some of these are pathogenic (associated with diseases), while others are very useful and necessary. Pasteur set out to prove that bacteria cause disease. To do this he isolated certain strains of bacteria in a sterile environment so he could study them scientifically. He also studied the effect of placing living organisms in a sterile environment and inoculating them with bacteria.

Now everyone knows that life can't exist in a sterile environment. If we sterilized everything that surrounds us, including the air, we would soon become very ill. This is especially true if we were to sterilize the internal environment of our intestines, since many of the bacteria which live there (the lactic acid bacteria) are essential for the synthesis of many life-supporting nutrients and vitamins.

On the ladder of evolution, bacteria are among the most primitive organisms. These microorganisms survive happily in a dead or decaying organism. Bacteria naturally invade a sterile environment and make it alive. Also, bacteria help dying material decompose back to a more primitive state. Since bacteria thrive as more complex life forms die, Pasteur's experiments were actually quite paradoxical. He studied the growth of bacteria in a sterile environment, and of course found that bacteria thrived and did very well; in fact, the bacteria spread.

By isolating specific strains of bacteria, Pasteur was able to develop what are known as antigens. An antigen is nothing more than a refined strain of pathogenic bacteria. This is what we are inoculated with when we are immunized. By injecting the antigen into our bodies we force the body to produce antibodies that defend us by attacking the invading bacterial strain. Specific antigens supposedly create immunity to specific diseases. This mechanism is the basis for the modern theory of immunization.

One of the problems with this idea is that vaccinations are designed to create an immunity to only one specific disease. The one particular antigen we are inoculated with produces antibodies that fight off a particular strain of bacteria. A broad immunity never develops, so a child may be vaccinated for measles and come down with mumps, or we might vaccinate for mumps and end up with a case of diphtheria. Modern medicine tries to meet this difficulty by increasing the number and variety of vaccinations, but its approach remains only a partial solution.

Remember that we live in an environment of germs. Germs are invading our body every moment of our lives; some of these germs are pathogenic. Since this is true, if germs are the cause of disease, then why aren't we fatally stricken from the moment we draw our first breath? How has the human species survived the many thousands of years that preceded the dawn of modern medicine?

Consider the interesting fact that many mothers have recently decided to give birth at home rather than in the hospital delivery room. It appears that the incidence of childhood sicknesses in the first two weeks after birth is much lower among infants born at home than among those born in the hospital. Common sense might tell us that the hospital is weakening these infants in some way and, in fact, it is the sterile environment of the delivery room that is to blame. In such an environment—an environment abnormally free of bacteria, the supposed cause of disease—the body is not forced to create any natural immunities to infection. Because the body is thus rendered defenseless, it easily sickens when removed from this artificial environment. If you have your baby at home, from the very first breath the child's body has begun to adapt itself to the world in which it will live—and it's also less likely to encounter the extremely serious bacteria and viruses that tend to collect in hospitals. The adaptability of the child is the key factor for health. Such adaptability cannot develop if the child remains in an artificial environment isolated from the healthy balance of nature.

Natural immunity is a response to the total environment in which we live. To be truly healthy, we cannot isolate our lives from that environment, nor can we single out any one aspect of the environment as the cause of our woes, as we seem to do with germs. We are only one part of a network that embraces all living things. To act as though we are special cases within this web of creation is actually to invite illness to appear. All such illness is only a symptom of our own imbalance. To be free of disease requires our developing a broad immunity. This can only happen in a balanced, natural environment.

An axiomatic procedure of modern science is to study isolated incidents rather than whole processes in their natural setting. Nature is seen as an interfering factor to be overcome. Modern medicine, along with other products of modern thinking, tends to view the world dualistically, in terms of "us against them." In our desire to understand sickness we have made germs the enemy; these tiny organisms must be isolated and destroyed—only then will humanity be free from disease! We scrub our hands before eating, sterilize our dishes after every meal, use more and more powerful soaps and detergents to clean things up. If people become seriously ill, then quick, put them in the sterilized hospital—seal off their environment, protect them from those horrible germs!

How often does anyone pause to consider the foolishness of this behavior? Actually, humanity is part of an extended network of creation that stretches back billions of years. Germs, or bacteria, were the beginning of life on this planet. They are the bridge between the world of atomic elements—inorganic matter—and the world of living things. If virus and bacteria had never "infected" this planet, we would not be here to worry about them today.

We should also realize that bacteria will only reproduce in damaged life. You can't grow miso on whole soybeans; you have to cook them and crush them before the bacteria will grow. The same idea applies to our blood. If our blood is strong and healthy, pathogenic bacteria will not reproduce in our body. The question is how to make ourselves stronger and more vital, not how to protect ourselves from bacteria and germs.

As our judgment improves and we learn to overcome many modern prejudices, we realize that it is impossible to alienate ourselves from this ancient, extended network of life. The modern desire to isolate oneself from the chain of creation is seen not only in the problem of immunization, but also in many of the assumptions that underlie our technological society. Much of our civilization is founded on the premise that we should isolate ourselves from each other and from the environment by owning separate automobiles, houses, bank accounts, and so forth. Modern medicine, with its radical, life-destroying treatments, is only a symptom of this mentality.

The macrobiotic approach is to embrace all aspects of our environment, to realize that our lives are a unity of the physical, mental, and spiritual worlds. We are not separate from the rest of creation but inseparably at one with it.

No other animal on earth worries about doctors and immunizations. Then again, no other species suffers from "the common cold," not to mention our degenerative diseases such as heart attacks, cancer, etc. Of course, no other animal has placed itself so far from the order of nature. What other animal weakens itself by eating food that has been chemically treated, processed, and adulterated—or tries to live in an extremely artificial environment filled with poisons?

As our unnatural lifestyle and diet continues to weaken our vitality, we grow sicker and worry more and more about medicine and the need for immunization against bacteria.

The simple truth is that bacteria are not really the cause of disease. Bacterial proliferation, which we call "infection," is one *result* of disease. It is a natural part of the process of decay. Sickness produces bacteria; bacteria do not cause disease.

Nevertheless, say the skeptics, hasn't it been proven that vaccinations have reduced the incidence of infectious disease? And what about polio?

Polio has gotten a lot of publicity over the past decades. Supporters of immunization often bring it out as a prime witness for their case. We've even made polio vaccination a legal requirement. How many vials of vaccine are sold to inoculate those millions of schoolchildren every year? Doctors may be very well-meaning, but their view of disease (in this particular case, polio) is to a large extent distorted by the research propaganda of the large pharmaceutical companies. Such companies of course have too much at stake to allow any nonbelievers to deny the ritual of vaccination. It's just not good business.

The significant fact is, however, that the incidence of polio began to rise around the 1940s, just when the consumption of highly refined foods such as white sugar and soda pop began spiralling upward towards astronomical figures and the traditional ways of American life were coming apart under the sway of post-war affluence. The obvious facts that polio was higher in the summer and highest in the Southern states, matching peaks of sugar and soft-drink consumption, were lost in the panicky warnings to avoid infection in public bathing places.

When responding to the question of polio we should also look at a study done in the late 1970's among the Pennsylvania Amish. These people have steadily resisted the government's efforts to inoculate them with anti-polio vaccine. The federal government, outraged at such heretical resistance to the modern religion of science, has sent word through its public health agencies in twenty-one states that citizens and schools should shun the Amish, since they are allegedly spreading a crippling disease. The health agencies claim that an "epidemic" has already broken out.

On closer examination, however, the facts are not quite so clear-cut. Dr. Robert Mendelsohn, in *The People's Doctor Newsletter*, points out that although four people have been diagnosed as "carrying" the polio virus, three of the "carriers" show no symptoms. He asks whether other groups have been tested to see if they are carriers without symptoms. Government doctors claim that the reason this "epidemic" broke out among the Amish is because they have not been vaccinated. Yet government statistics reveal that approximately one-third of all schoolchildren in this country have not been vaccinated. Why hasn't the polio virus chosen to pick on any of those other children who do not share the heretical Amish views about official science?

Doctors commonly cite the declining incidence of infectious diseases as proof for their assumption that vaccinations are doing their job. As Ivan Illich's book, *Medical Nemesis* (Pantheon, 1976), makes clear, these statistics are quite misleading. The decline in certain diseases was caused by factors of lifestyle, such as sanitation, which had no direct connection to the increase in immunization. In addition to *Medical Nemesis*, books such as Bernard Dixson's *Beyond the Magic Bullet* (Harper & Row, 1978) and Robert Mendelsohn's *Confessions of a Medical Heretic* (Contemporary Books, 1979) also point out that the incidence of infectious disease was already in a declining course before vaccination became widespread.

In general, modern society, through its increasing artificiality, tends to inhibit the outbreak of infectious diseases. The infectious diseases—with their symptoms of fever, skin rashes or pustules, diarrhea, and so forth—are nothing but methods of discharge which the body undergoes to maintain balance. Modern society, by encouraging an overly protective lifestyle, prevents these symptoms from occurring, to our detriment later on. The paralysis associated with polio, for example, is caused by the overconsumption of yin foods such as sugar and chemicals, particularly when taken in a cold form as in soft drinks. Polio began to appear when various childhood diseases of discharge had been suppressed by modern medications such as penicillin. Although the specific symptoms we call polio may be suppressed, the undischarged accumulation of excess yin may take on even more serious forms, such as cancer, later on.

Researchers, however, in their quest for criminals and culprits in the forms of viruses and bacteria will not tolerate such commonsense explanations. Even though the World Health Organization has recently stated that we spend too much time and money chasing germs and not enough improving our own vitality as the best defense against sickness through better diet and nutrition, doctors still proclaim that vaccinations are a cure-all for our woes.

If disease is not caused by bacteria, then who shall we blame? We must learn to understand symptoms and their origin so we can adjust our diet and lifestyle to restore our natural immunity to disease. Only by understanding sickness will we be able to assume responsibility for our health and decrease our dependence on modern medicine.

Childhood Fevers
Keeping Your Cool When Temperatures Rise

by BARBARA AND LEONARD JACOBS

W aking up in the middle of the night to take care of your crying child, you realize the problem might be serious. The child is hot and sweaty—feverish—yet complaining of being cold. She seems to be trembling and you wonder if convulsions are about to develop. You feel helpless and worried. Should you call a doctor or try something on your own?

The onset of a fever in a small child is often a traumatic time for parents. We have been conditioned to think that fever is an indication of a major problem and are immediately tempted to find an expert who can help us bring it down. Should a pediatrician or some other health professional who knows more than us be given the responsibility?

Over the years, we have been asked more frequently about how to deal with fevers than about any other childhood problem. Yet fevers can usually be treated quite simply by parents. In fact, in the past few years, most conventional health practitioners have begun to agree that a fever in itself is not really a very serious problem. Fever, they now say, is a key element in the body's system of defense—an ally against invading organisms. "The evidence that fever is in and of itself an important defense mechanism is mounting rapidly," says Dr. Paul S. Lietman, professor of medicine, pediatrics, and pharmacology at Johns Hopkins Medical School in Baltimore. "Its action is directed against both bacterial infections and viruses." Dr. David Lang, chief of pediatrics at the University of Maryland School of Medicine, claims, "The concept that fever, especially in children, desperately demands eradication is totally erroneous. The body is wiser than we. We shouldn't interfere with normal body responses to illness, just because we have the ability to do so." Even convulsions, which can develop in young children from the rapid rise in body temperature, are not really dangerous and do not cause brain damage.

By understanding fevers one can understand childhood health problems in general. A fever is also an opportunity for parents to decide whether they are able to be their child's own "doctor" or whether they want to have some other "expert" advise them. It is possible to treat fevers at home with simple food preparations, teas, and compresses. The essential thing to know is: What caused the fever? Is the underlying cause serious enough to require special treatment, or is it merely a healthy reaction to some imbalance in the child?

After discussing the general nature and mechanisms of a fever and its possible causes, we will explain some of the preparations used in treating it. With all the facts at hand, you will be better prepared to make a thoughtful decision in a calm atmosphere.

The Nature of Fever

Fever is the body's response to some internal imbalance, of dietary or environmental origin. For instance, when the body becomes overly acidic or alkaline, the thyroid often responds by increasing the metabolic rate and raising the body temperature. Also, when an infection is detected by the body's immune system, certain white blood cells are activated to deal with it, and a fever results. The activated blood cells instigate the release of a hormone called endogenous pyrogen ("endogenous" signifies that it is made within the body; "pyrogen" is derived from the Greek word meaning "fire-producer"), which travels through the bloodstream to the brain. In the brain, this hormone acts on the hypothalamus (a tiny structure located near the intersection of the spinal cord and the brain), which regulates body temperature like a thermostat. After it receives the hormone's message, the hypothalamus sets a new temperature for the body. The body responds with chills, which force it to raise its temperature to the new setting. In addition, outlying blood vessels are constricted to reduce heat loss, and body tissues such as stored fat are broken down to produce more heat. Nerve messages trigger rapid muscle contractions, or shivering, which helps to produce even more heat. (Endogenous pyrogen also reduces the level of iron in the blood, an element which is necessary for the development of infectious bacteria and viruses.)

In these two instances, fever is simply the body's automatic response to an imbalanced condition. There are, of course, some symptoms which indicate the necessity of taking the fever more seriously. If the fever stays around 101.5 degrees F. for more than a day, or if it lasts for four or more days, regardless of how high it is, it may signal that a more serious condition is the underlying cause. In addition, a fever of over 104 degrees F. should not be allowed to run for more than a few hours without some kind of treatment.

Meningitis, a rare condition sometimes associated with high or persistent fevers, is an infection of the meninges (the fluid surrounding the spinal cord), which can travel to the brain and possibly cause brain damage. When our first child, Jesse, was eight months old, he had a fever of 103.5 degrees. We used all the remedies we knew of to treat it, but after being unable to reduce it after twenty-four hours, we went to a pediatrician. He gave our son one teaspoon of "temperin" (a form of aspirin for children) and within one hour the temperature went down to 99 degrees. Although he recommended continuing the dosage for another twenty-four hours, we gave Jesse only one more teaspoonful and have never had to use any other medication for him since. He is now twelve years old. We had been concerned about the possibility of meningitis in our son's case, as this is one serious (though uncommon) condition which can develop by allowing a fever of over 104 degrees to continue for more than a few hours without treatment. Pneumonia could also be indicated by a fever of this type.

Aspirin

The ancient Greeks regarded disease as an imbalance of "humors." They believed fever cooked the bad humors and helped the body to get rid of them. In the Orient there was a similar belief that fever was the body's natural response to some unbalanced condition—the mechanism that brought into balance the natural harmony of "yin and yang." The notion that fever was beneficial persisted for more than 2,000 years and countless patients were actually treated with "fever therapy" to aid their recovery from such ailments as syphilis, tuberculosis, and even hysteria. Then, in the mid-1800s, aspirin compounds that rapidly reduced fevers became commercially available and the medical view of fever changed abruptly. For the next 100 years, physicians and patients focused on bringing down fevers, sometimes with pharmaceuticals and sometimes with other therapies.

Recent studies support the view of the Greek and Oriental peoples. It seems that fever may have evolved at least 300 million years ago in cold-blooded vertebrates as a means of fighting invading organisms. These new findings raise serious questions about the wisdom of taking aspirin for fevers below 104 degrees. In fact, a number of pediatricians are now suggesting that moderate fevers be allowed to run their course, as they may shorten the illness and reduce the possibility of spreading infection to other people. In addition, aspirin may actually interfere with the body's natural fight against viruses for the same reason that it brings down the fever. Aspirin blocks the output of prostaglandins—hormones which raise the temperature but which also allow interferon and lysozymes (the body's natural antiviral substances) to act. Aspirin has also been implicated in the development of Reye's Syndrome, a rare but potentially fatal condition that has been reported to occur most often after the onset of a viral illness which is then treated with aspirin. Both the U.S. Surgeon General, C. Everett Koop, and the American Academy of Pediatrics' Committee on Infectious Diseases, advise that children should not take aspirin or any other medications containing salicylates (the major ingredient of aspirin) in treating the common flu or chicken pox.

Home Treatments

Most of us recall the recommendation to "starve a fever." This old adage may be incorrect. Rather than starving a fever, it may be best to feed it. Some foods you may want to give your child are soft-cooked whole grain cereals, mild miso soup, lightly steamed greens, and boiled tofu with a small amount of tamari and fresh ginger. These foods are nourishing while being very mild, and they will not exaggerate any other nutritional imbalance. Make sure that your child has plenty of liquids and does not become dehydrated, since that is one of the effects of a fever.

Make the child comfortable and observe him or her closely. It may not be necessary to take the temperature more than twice a day although you will want to have a general idea of how high it actually is. You can take the temperature either with a rectal or an oral thermometer although the rectal thermometer will register a temperature one degree higher than the oral one. With an oral thermometer, you can also take the temperature by holding it under the armpit for four minutes.

With children under one year old, you may need to apply some treatment if the temperature gets above 103 degrees. And regardless of the age, you may have to use some sort of treatment if the temperature stays at 104 or higher for more than four hours. However, it is usually not necessary to use any type of medication unless a fever this high persists for more than 24 hours. A fever is generally higher in the late afternoon and evening, lower in the morning. You can tell when a fever is about to break (that is, to go down) when it does not go up in the late afternoon. Sweating is the other indication that a fever is about to break. This happens because the body is naturally cooling itself as a way to bring the fever down.

Be sure that the child's underwear and bedclothes are made of cotton, which absorbs sweat better than synthetics. Also, unless the child has the chills, do not bundle him or her up since this will prevent sweat from evaporating and keep the body temperature too high. Sponging the child with a cool washcloth may be necessary if he or she is very uncomfortable. And if the fever does reach 104 degrees or more, you can put the child in a lukewarm or cool bath in order to lower the body temperature. Another treatment which is very effective is to place a cool washcloth or crushed lettuce or cabbage leaves on the forehead while at the same time placing the feet in warm water—this will re-establish the natural balance of coolness at the top of the body, warmth at the bottom.

A tofu plaster is often effective in reducing fevers. Tofu, a soybean product, is available in most natural foods stores and Oriental markets and increasingly in regular supermarkets. Take half a tofu cake, or approximately six ounces, and squeeze out the excess liquid. Mix this with a small amount of flour and freshly grated ginger and place in a piece of cheesecloth. You can then apply this mixture to the back of the child's neck or behind the ears as a way of cooling the head and reducing the fever.

While treating the fever, observe whether or not the child continues to have daily bowel movements. If she or he is constipated, there is stagnation in the intestines which may be breeding the infection. In order to eliminate this stagnation, you should try to get the child to continue eating, even if only soups and soft cereals. If the child has no appetite, is constipated, and continues to be feverish, you may have to give an enema of lukewarm bancha tea.

Recommended beverages while treating the fever are water, bancha or kukicha tea with or without lemon, and diluted apple juice. A preparation which is very effective in stimulating urination--called a diuretic--is tea made from the juice of freshly grated daikon (or icicle) radish. Simply wash the unpeeled radish, grate it fairly finely, squeeze the juice through cheesecloth and heat this liquid (approximately 3 to 4 ounces) in a small saucepan. You can add a few drops of tamari or a few grains of sea salt for flavor. Radish drink may have a very sharp, strong taste so you may be able to give the child only several drops, but even that small amount can be effective in inducing sweating and stimulating urination. This treatment is recommended only if the child's fever is over 103 or 104 and he or she is uncomfortable and has no appetite. Otherwise you may simply allow the fever to run its course, which may take an average of eighteen hours.

It may seem difficult to ride out the fever and not overreact. But if you can be responsive and attentive, this may be the best way to learn about your child's inner balances and allow him or her to heal without outside interference. Childhood sicknesses are not "bad." In most instances, they are opportunities for the children to develop their own identities and personalities in response to natural and simple causes. You may have to spend more time in dealing with your child than you would if you were treating with medication, but the result will be worth the extra effort.

Choosing a Doctor

Parents may have to consider, when treating a child's fever, when to call in an outside professional. If the parents do not have the time—or lack the confidence—to deal with the fever themselves, it may be necessary to ask another parent or professional for advice. We recommend making friends with a health professional as soon as possible to call on in case of need. Even though you might be able to treat many childhood ailments yourself, it may be necessary to go to a pediatrician, naturopath, or homeopath for routine physicals in preparation for admission to public schools. You also may have to consult with a pediatrician regarding the issue of childhood immunizations which are often required for your child to enter school. Rather than isolating yourself from medical doctors, we feel it is best to search out doctors who are sympathetic to, or understanding of, your point of view.

If you do not already know a medical doctor, you may want to consider the following questions when interviewing prospective health professionals. Questions like these will allow you to evaluate the doctors and understand their perspective on health care in general:

1. *How do you feel about natural childbirth?*
2. *Do you routinely administer all childhood immunizations?*
3. *How do you feel about tonsillectomies?*
4. *For what ailments do you suggest using medications?*
5. *What would you use for a fever?*
6. *What are your thoughts on circumcision?*
7. *Do you make house calls, or do you ever see patients outside of usual office hours?*
8. *Where are you continuing your professional studies?*

The answers to these kinds of questions will give you some idea of the sensitivity of the health professional to the total well-being of your child. Although there are no "right" answers, if the doctor routinely uses medications and surgical procedures, you will know what to expect when your child is being treated.

You can often find sensitive, sympathetic, and responsible medical doctors at holistic health centers, community health care clinics, and at some teaching hospitals. We have found that physicians who travel to Third World countries for study and fieldwork are the most sensitive to the overall health of the child. These professionals are the least likely to use the most modern therapies and at the same time are usually the most knowledgeable about the use of alternative and folk remedies. At some point you may have to trust this person completely—allowing the health professional to exercise his or her best judgment even though the treatment may appear fairly extreme. After all, this is the reason you have gone to a doctor, and you will have to give up a certain amount of personal involvement for the long-term benefit of the child.

Treating Childhood Ailments
How the Body Adjusts to the Seasons

BY BARBARA AND LEONARD JACOBS

A balanced and healthy pregnancy and a good diet for your child do not mean that she or he won't become sick periodically. In fact, if the child does not develop some minor symptoms when the seasons change you may want to find some way to encourage these fluctuations by giving her or him either more salty food (if the previous season was summer) or fruit (if it was winter). The reason for this is that even someone who is living in harmony with the environment invariably takes in some excess which will manifest itself when the weather changes. It is practically impossible to eat and live in total harmony with the current season and at the same time be prepared for the new one. For instance, during the hot days of summer your child may eat large amounts of salad or fruit. Often this may be too much for the cold weather in the fall, so the child may get a runny nose or cold as a way of adjusting to the new season.

Around the time of the equinoxes and solstices, therefore, you can expect some minor health problems. Rather than being alarmed you should regard these symptoms as a sign of resilience and flexibility. The child is naturally making adjustments, and rarely are there any complications from these types of ailments. The most common symptoms are runny nose, cough, diarrhea, constipation, tonsillitis, or other swollen lymph glands.

If you are able to encourage the child's adjustment through these symptoms and at the same time prevent a high fever, there should be no problem. You may have to discriminate between yin and yang conditions. Yin conditions generally appear as swellings, skin eruptions, mild fevers, frequent urination, diarrhea, head colds, sore throats, and emotional irritability. Yang sicknesses are characterized by high fevers, constipation, dry coughing, redness, and outbursts of anger. Generally you can treat yin sicknesses with yang preparations and yang sicknesses with yin preparations.

In many cases a child's condition may be from an excess of yin and yang simultaneously. One simple method to determine whether the child needs yin (fruit, liquid, and so forth) or yang (salt or baked food) is to give the child a choice of the two extremes. For example, allow her or him to choose between a fresh apple and daikon pickle or a bowl of miso soup. If the child chooses both she or he may actually need both. Basic yin medicinal preparations are: warm fruit juice, apple or pear sauce, rice malt, grated fresh apple with a few drops of tamari soy sauce, grated fresh ginger in bancha tea, amesake, and daikon radish drink. You may invent other treatments depending on what is available in your kitchen and based on what you feel may have been the cause of the child's sickness. For instance, if the child has been visiting friends and ate more animal food than she or he is used to eating, you may want to make some fresh orange juice or grapefruit juice as a way of re-establishing balance.

Yang preparations to balance yin conditions include miso soup, a few drops of tamari soy sauce in bancha tea, mild mu tea, brine or bran pickles, umeboshi plum in bancha tea, roasted umeboshi powder, lotus root tea, and kuzu with umeboshi, tamari, and ginger. Some preparations which are a combination of yin and yang include kuzu with fruit juice or rice malt, steamed or sautéed leafy vegetables, bancha tea with lemon or rice malt, baked tempeh with mustard, cooked seaweed with tamari soy sauce, and a tea made from the liquid left over when cooking hiziki or arame. One additional food which is often effective in treating a child who is experiencing both yin and yang symptoms is a piece of kombu left over from making kombu stock.

You will naturally have to use your judgment in deciding which preparation is suitable for your child's condition. The choice depends on her or his constitution, as well as the time of year and the primary cause of the symptoms. You should remember that approximately 90 percent of all children's sicknesses will be cured with no treatment except time. The body has an inherent ability to heal itself and should receive a minimum of interference. Try to keep a positive image about your child's health. Keep her or him mildly stimulated with play or some games. Within a day or two the child should recover. If the treatment was appropriate, the child's health will be even stronger than before.

In any case, we can and should expect our children to "get sick" periodically, but these temporary discharges can help create greater resistance and flexibility. Difficulties of all types can serve as stimuli for self-reflection and as opportunities, for both us and our children, to develop judgment. When symptoms such as fevers, swellings, coughs, and rashes appear, we can encourage our children to relate the "sickness" to some specific imbalance in their diet or environment. They can thus begin to learn the importance of their daily diet and lifestyle in establishing their own health. Experiencing problems is one of the best ways to learn how to solve problems and to understand the causes and effects of our interaction with the environment.

Understanding and Treating Childhood Sicknesses

Yin sicknesses are generally caused by excessive consumption of yin (sweet, juicy, spicy) foods and appear as swellings, skin eruptions, mild fevers, frequent urination, diarrhea, and emotional irritability. Head colds, sore throats, swollen glands, and tuberculosis are all yin— caused by too much yin food.

Yang sicknesses, on the other hand, are caused by excessive consumption of yang (salty, dry, chewy) foods and appear as emotional tightness, high fevers, redness, constipation, and outbursts of anger. Thus, measles, pneumonia, dry coughing, and appendicitis are all yang.

The scientific names of sicknesses are only arbitrary labels for various gradations of the two general categories of sickness. I will briefly describe the conventional symptomatology of the most common childhood sicknesses.

Many children's illnesses are related to the lymph system and often are caused by accumulation of excess mucus. This mucus can result from eating sugar, fatty foods (such as milk, cheese, and yogurt), and white flour, or by overeating in general. By noting the area of the body affected and the types of food your child has been eating, you can usually figure out the dietary cause of the sickness. For instance, eating sugar creates an acidic condition in the blood, which at first causes skin problems and sluggish intestines—either constipation or diarrhea. Milk creates mucus in the throat and lungs, causing coughing, sneezing, and a runny nose. If you have no success in diagnosing and treating your child, don't be afraid to consult an expert of your choice, whether that be a pediatrician, acupuncturist, or naturopath. Consulting such experts offers us excellent opportunities to develop our own judgment, if we use our time with them to learn.

Chicken pox is a very common childhood sickness, occurring most often in the winter and spring. The symptoms begin with a fever, which rarely goes above 101-102 degrees. A rash of pink blotches appears late on the first day or on the second day of illness. In the center of the pink spots, tiny blisters appear which continue to come out fresh each day, as the blotches increase in number, all over the body. The blisters may itch, and if scratched and broken they may leave small scars. In view of these symptoms, chicken pox is a yin sickness, usually caused by drinking too much citrus fruit and juices in the colder months of the year.

Diphtheria (a relatively rare disease in the U.S.) is characterized by a sore throat, mild fever, and possibly the development of a membrane covering the throat. This membrane may remain for seven or eight days and can make breathing difficult. The serious complications include heart failure and temporary paralysis of the limbs and respiratory muscles. Diphtheria is a yin sickness, and its usual cause is heavy consumption of rich dairy foods, fruits, and sugar.

German measles (Rubella) is a common childhood disease. The symptoms are mild: fever, swollen lymph nodes behind the ear or at the back of the head, and often a rash of flat, pink spots. This disease is considered serious only for women in the first three months of pregnancy: It was discovered that 20 percent of such women had babies with birth defects. German measles is also a yin disease, caused by excessive consumption of raw vegetables out of season and nonregional fruits.

Measles (Rubeola) is a very common childhood sickness which begins like a common cold. The symptoms—a hard, dry cough, irritated eyes, and high fever—usually appear on the second day. A rash appears on the third or fourth day, beginning behind the ears or at the hairline and spreading downward, covering the entire body in about thirty-six hours. The rash begins with small pink spots, which often run together into itchy blotches. Measles usually reaches its peak of intensity on the sixth day; it then subsides within a few days. Measles is a yang disease, and it usually develops only once in a child; it can be seen as a natural discharge of excess yang accumulated in the embryological stage from the mother. This natural discharge should not be suppressed, since it is part of the process of growth involved in normal full maturation of the physical and mental faculties. This disease is best treated by keeping the child away from excessive stimulation, in a dark, humid, quiet room, and feeding very mild foods such as rice cream.

Mumps, another common childhood disease, begins with a fever of 100-102 degrees, headache, and fatigue. Within two days one or both of the salivary glands in front of the ears becomes swollen, and it may be painful to swallow. The entire illness usually lasts only five or six days. This is a yin disease, caused by consumption of fatty animal foods and especially dairy foods of all kinds.

Whooping cough (Pertussis) is a fairly common children's sickness. It usually begins as cold symptoms, followed by three to six weeks of violent coughing. The cough is "hacking" in the beginning and is fairly frequent. As the sickness progresses, the coughing comes in spells, occurring three or four times during the day or night. The coughing is an attempt to get rid of thick mucus, which often is partially discharged in the intense bouts of coughing. This yin sickness is caused by salty cheeses and milk.

Tetanus (or "lockjaw") is a disease caused by a puncture wound that does not bleed. The risk of acquiring tetanus is one in 600,000 in the U.S., and 73 percent of reported cases in 1974 occurred in people over the age of fifty. The symptoms of tetanus begin with stiffness of the muscles in the jaw and neck. Within two days muscle rigidity may have spread to the torso and limbs; the body may become "stiff as a board." The conventional treatment for this disease is very drastic. Tetanus is a yin disease which can usually be avoided by seeing that your child develops a strong physical constitution and by making certain that any deep puncture wound bleeds.

Poliomyelitis (polio) is a very rare disease which begins with symptoms similar to a cold or the flu but is often followed by stiffness of the back and neck and muscle pain. Paralysis of the arms and/or legs may occur next. Predisposing factors to polio include recent tonsillectomy, immunizations, and tooth extractions. Polio is a yin disease, caused by consumption of refined foods, citrus fruits, and sugar. It is more common in the summer and in the Southern states, where greater quantities of modern-style yin foods (such as soft drinks and ice cream) are consumed.

The common cold is a mild sickness characterized by sneezing, low fever, runny nose, and headaches. The constant discharge of mucus associated with a cold indicates that it is a yin sickness caused by consumption of sweet foods and dairy foods.

Besides eliminating the foods indicated for each individual sickness, an effective method for treating, as well as preventing, childhood sicknesses is to provide a well-balanced diet of grains, vegetables, sea vegetables, beans, and nuts. A sensible introduction to this diet is available in *The Book of Macrobiotics* by Michio Kushi (New York: Japan Publications, 1977).

Short term treatments can also be very effective, and in my experience ginger compresses, mustard plasters, kuzu tea, and massage can help to ease the symptoms of childhood sicknesses. For skin problems and rashes, ginger compresses on the kidneys and rice or chlorophyll plasters on the skin are most effective. For respiratory ailments, lotus root tea and mustard plasters work especially well. For digestive problems, ginger compresses on the intestines and kuzu tea with an umeboshi plum, tamari soy sauce, and fresh grated ginger root can be very beneficial. For fevers, use daikon tea.

Some other problems which you may experience with your child are burns, cuts, and poisoning. Of course if your child gets a serious burn you had better go to a professional medical person, but for minor burns immediately wash the area with cold salt water. This should prevent blistering. If the burn is still painful apply tofu or aloe vera gel and cover with gauze or cheesecloth. Avoid fruit juices or citrus fruit for several days after the burn to accelerate the healing. For a cut which doesn't require stitches, first be sure that it has bled. Puncture wounds which don't bleed can lead to tetanus. Then wash the cut with salt water and if it is still bleeding cover with diluted miso and then with cheesecloth or gauze. (The enzymes in the miso promote rapid healing.) For poisoning, especially by acidic-type substances such as paint, gasoline, and chemicals, give the child warm salt water and induce vomiting. In many cases, however, you may need to contact the poison center or medical doctor in your area for further help with antidotes.

Recipes for Special Treatment

All medicinal preparations are best made in glass dishes or earthenware pots; metal pots may contaminate these foods with unwanted elements and may interact with the preparations to defeat their purpose.

Daikon Tea

Take a small daikon root or a piece about six to eight inches long, grate it, and squeeze out the juice. Heat up the juice until it is just beginning to boil, then add a couple of drops of tamari soy sauce so its taste is only mildly sharp. After taking daikon tea the child should stay warm, preferably in bed. This will encourage sweating and urination and will also help bring down a fever.

Kuzu With Rice Malt

For colds, fever, and headaches, thoroughly dissolve approximately one to one-and-a-half tablespoons of kuzu in one cup of cool water. Heat this up, stirring continuously, until it begins to look translucent. Add two to three tablespoons of rice malt to make a fairly thick and sweet custard. This drink is best taken while it's still warm.

Umeshoyu Kuzu (kuzu with umeboshi, tamari, and ginger)

Thoroughly dissolve one to one-and-a-half tablespoons of kuzu in a cup of cold water. While heating this up, add the pieces of one umeboshi plum. As the kuzu begins to thicken add one-eighth to one-fourth teaspoon of grated fresh ginger and several drops of tamari soy sauce. Kuzu can be used for indigestion and other intestinal problems and colds.

Lotus Root Tea

This tea, especially good for coughs and other lung and respiratory problems, is made by grating a medium-sized (4 to 6 inches), firm, washed lotus root and squeezing out the juice. Add equal amounts of spring water to the lotus root juice and heat this mixture over a medium flame until it thickens. You can then add a small amount of fresh grated ginger and a few drops of tamari for flavor.

Mustard Plaster

One other treatment that's especially effective for young children who have coughs or lung congestion is a mustard plaster. This is made by mixing approximately two tablespoons of fresh dried mustard with two to three tablespoons of water. The mixture should be a smooth and slightly runny paste. Take a piece of waxed paper and spread the mixture over half of it. Fold the paper in half, and seal up the edges so that none of the mixture oozes out. Place a thin towel on the lung area of the child and put the mustard plaster on top. Cover with another towel. The skin under this plaster will begin to get quite hot in about 20 minutes. Be sure to take off the mustard plaster as soon as the skin begins to get hot in order to prevent the skin from burning. You could continue to use the same mustard plaster for several days repeating the application once every several hours.

Ginger Compress

Pour 4 pints of water into an enamel pot with a close-fitting lid, cover place on the stove and bring to a boil. Meanwhile grate the unpeeled ginger and place it in the cotton sack, which is tied off. When the water has come to a boil, turn off the heat. Wait until the water has ceased boiling, squeeze the sack of ginger so the juice runs into the water, place the sack in the pot, and replace the lid. It is very important that the ginger is not placed in the pot while the water is boiling as this will markedly reduce the effectiveness of the treatment. The same water can be used for three or four treatments. Fold towels so that they are four to six inches wide, and immerse them so that the edges are dry and the bulk of the towel is in the ginger water. When thoroughly soaked, remove, squeeze excess liquid back into the pot, and replace the lid. The area of skin over the organ you wish to treat should be exposed. The person being treated should be lying in a comfortable, relaxed position. The towels are then placed so they cover the area of treatment completely. It is preferable to use two layers of towels. These are then covered with the bath towel, which helps to keep the heat in. The temperature of the hot, soaked towels should be as warm as the person being treated can stand, but not so hot that they burn. Leave the hot towels in place until cool, then repeat the procedure until the skin becomes red. Try to keep the temperature of the skin constant. The treatment should last for approximately half an hour; you will know it is working when the patient's skin becomes reddened.

Chlorophyll Plaster

A chlorophyll plaster is made by mashing fresh greens, such as lettuce or cabbage in a suribachi or mortar. It should be applied directly behind the child's ears.

Tofu Plaster

A tofu plaster is squeezed tofu mixed with about 15 to 20 percent white flour and a small amount of grated fresh ginger. It should be wrapped in cheesecloth and applied behind the ears as with the chlorophyll plaster.

Rice Plaster

A rice plaster is prepared by mashing three parts cooked brown rice in a suribachi together with one part raw green leafy vegetables and one part untoasted nori seaweed. Apply directly to skin. This treatment is very good for boils.

A complete list of symptomatic treatments is given in *The Book of Macrobiotics* by Michio Kushi, *Zen Macrobiotics* by Georges Ohsawa, and *Healing Ourselves* by Noboru Muramoto (New York: Avon Books, 1977). I also recommend the following organizations and publications for information and ideas on childhood sicknesses and immunizations: The American Vegan Society (501 Old Harding Highway, Malaga, NJ 08328); Sheltrano Hygiean Paradise, Inc. (Drawer X, Keystone Rd., Pearsall, TX 78061); East West Foundation (P.O. Box 850, Brookline, MA 02146); *Immunizations: Are They Necessary?* by Randy Neustaedter (Hering Family Health Clinic, Suite 107, 2340 Ward St., Berkeley, CA 94905); *Don't Get Stuck* by Hannah Allen (Healthways Publications, Keystone Rd., Pearsall, TX 78061); *How to Raise a Healthy Child in Spite of Your Doctor* by Robert Mendelsohn, M.D., (Contemporary Books, Chicago, IL); *Immunology,* by David Gray (Edward Arnold Publishers, London); *When Your Child is Ill,* by Samuel Karelits, M.D. (Natural Hygiene Press, 1920 W. Irving Park Rd., Chicago, IL 60613); *Vegetarian World,* September 1977 (8235 Santa Monica Blvd., Los Angeles, CA 90046).

The steps in healing your children's sicknesses are first, to understand the real cause of the sickness; second, to adjust your child's diet; and third, to administer specific treatments. You should remember that childhood illnesses usually are indications of children's ability to discharge excess and are signs of their basic health and vitality.

Healthy Nutrition

Children and Junk Food
What To Do When Your Child Is Exposed To Unhealthy Foods

BY ANNEMARIE COLBIN

Bringing a child up in a world of soft drinks, candy bars, and mass-produced hamburgers is no easy task. In thousands of households, convincing children to eat homemade bread, vegetable soup, and bean salad is a problem receiving increasing attention.

My children are now eight and twelve years old. They grew up with brown rice cereal, steamed vegetables, and cooked beans. They relished, and still do, miso soup and nori seaweed, raw celery and carrots, and fresh fruit. They especially love green salad with lemon, tamari, and olive oil dressing—a dressing into which they also like to dip artichoke leaves. You may have guessed already the problem I faced as they grew older and left home more often: Friends in school teased them about their lunches, well-meaning adults offered them candy and milk, and pervasive junk food messages barked at them from the TV.

When my oldest daughter was going to nursery school, there was a spate of birthday parties with their attendant "treats." After several untouched lunches (would you want to eat lunch at 12:30 if you'd had cupcakes with icing at 11:00?), I decided it was time to do something. So I wrote an "Open Letter to Parents and Teachers" (see at end of article). I stood at the school door and handed out copies of my letter to the parents and teachers of my daughter's class. A few days later, the administration called to reprimand me for doing such an irregular thing—even though they agreed with me. But I didn't mind the ruffled feathers, because the results were more than I had dared to hope for; cupcakes virtually disappeared from the classroom, and parents started sending raisins and bananas whenever there was a birthday party.

Schools are often responsive to the personal involvement of parents concerned about nutrition. And even in 1974, when I wrote my letter, some mothers confessed that they were aware of good nutrition but didn't feel enough support to make changes. Today, with the public's increasing nutritional awareness, more and more people are willing to listen.

All parents who have been raising their children on a vegetarian or whole foods diet eventually have to face the problem of "outside" food. Most of us have discovered that the worst thing we can do is be harsh and unyielding in our prohibitions and thus instill fear and guilt in our children.

Guilt, as we all know, breeds lying, stealth, and sneakiness. Is that what we want our children to learn? Long ago, I decided that I didn't. When my daughter went to a school which included lunch, I knew I was faced with a fateful choice: Either she ate my food and found herself singled out as the only kid with a lunch bag, or she threw it out and sneaked school food, or I removed pressure and just let her have the lunch. I opted for the latter and decided to take an attitude that Wendy Wollner, another Boston mother, also found useful: minimize the importance of school lunch. "I look at their lunches as a snack," Wendy said, "and make sure that they have something more substantial when they get home." In addition, I started preparing breakfast meals: soup, vegetables, grain, and sometimes beans. I figured that if she had a good start in the morning, lunch wouldn't be such a crucial event.

The experiment was worth it. Shana ate the school lunch and wasn't any the worse for it, except that she did get her one and only cavity, thanks to the desserts—usually fruit, but canned in syrup. I was in fact thrilled with that cavity. Now she knew I was right when I said that sugar was bad for the teeth! Her own experience had told her only that candy tasted good and she had been unable to understand why Mommy would not let her eat it.

Our next adventure with candy happened when she became old enough for an allowance. "This is my money?" she asked. I said yes. "Can I buy anything I want with it?" I cleared my throat and said, "Yes, sort of." "Can I buy candy with it?" was the inevitable next question. "Well," I hesitated, torn between fairness and parental concern over health, "I guess you can, but I wish you wouldn't."

Unfortunately, I had always wanted my children to be strong, fearless though sensible, independent and confident. Now I was getting what I had asked for. "I'm going to buy candy," she decided. I felt it was more important to let her feel what it meant to make a personal choice than to break her will and make her obey me. Sooner or later, she would be old enough to be reasoned with. So for the next three months I let her spend her allowance trying out every candy bar on the market (except for green, red, or blue gumballs). Some friends who share my general dietary philosophy did not approve of my condoning this "research." I think they felt that once she had tasted all those candy bars she would be doomed to sugar addiction and would turn her back on good food forever.

Nothing of the sort happened. After three months, I suggested that it might be time to end the experiment. She agreed immediately and has shown no more interest in commercial candy bars since then. An occasional "Yinnie" candy or fruit bar from the health food store keeps her quite happy.

Alert parents soon realize that the problem is not food, but socialization. "Sharing of food is one of the prime social contacts," stated the government report, *Dietary Goals for the United States.* The wonderful food that we provide at home for our children isolates them socially; they cannot understand why their peers will ridicule what their parents so strongly approve of. They are placed in a very conflicting situation with, on the one hand, loving and perhaps stern parents giving them food that's kind of nice but not always colorful or exciting, and on the other hand, friends who eat stuff that tastes quite interesting and often appears on TV. Healthy children are curious and they continually explore the world around them. Can we blame them for wanting to try things? It would be to the benefit of us all if we made a real effort to understand the serious conflict our children are in with food and to try to ease it somewhat.

For socialization, the question of sharing is paramount. Wendy Wollner found that her seven-year-old son was delighted to offer his guests familiar foods like fruit juices, fruit, whole grain cookies, and rice cakes. My kids decided to buck the disapproval of their friends and take rice balls to school anyway because they liked them. Soon I was making extras for their friends, and nori-wrapped brown rice balls with a bit of umeboshi paste at the center became a hot item in school. The sharing can go both ways: Our children's friends can share our food but we must also allow our children to share their friends' food once in a while, regardless of quality. I'm convinced that love transcends "bad" food.

Therefore, my kids are allowed to eat anything they want when they go to a birthday party. I considered letting them take along some "wholesome" treats but rejected that as an implied criticism of the hosts which would not, I felt, go unnoticed. Instead, I try to stuff them beforehand. At first, I tried hearty foods like kasha or bean soup, but I realized that they would eat more sweets to counterbalance. Then I opted for offering them homemade sweets and fruit before they went to the party; this way they are less interested in additional sweets.

With regard to packing school lunches, I discovered what many other parents also found out—we have to communicate with the children, ask their opinion, and provide them with the kind of good food that they will eat. Recently, for example, I noticed that Kaila, my eight-year-old, began to return her thermos unopened. After consulting with her and watching what she ate and what she didn't eat, I noticed that the thermos food was generally in disfavor, unless it was soup. When I gave her more individual, separate foods, that she could eat by hand, such as sesame butter sandwiches, carrot sticks, cucumbers, fruit, and so on, her lunch appeared more "normal" and she ate it without protest.

Next to communication, the most important thing is honesty, following our principles consistently, and not having dietary double standards. I have a weakness for croissants (and there are four croissant shops within six blocks of my home) so of course the children can have croissants once a week as I do. And they know that there is a choice in matters of food. While I don't eat meat, my husband does, once in a while. Shana has already informed me that she doesn't think she'll be a vegetarian when she grows up—an interesting comment, since while I was pregnant with her, all I craved was animal protein, including meat. (Did I eat it? Yes, some, but not as much as I wanted.) As a hungry pre-teen, she indeed does well if she consumes some tunafish or chicken two or three times a week but she has also discovered that too much meat gives her nightmares.

All that I hope for is that my children learn that food is important for our well-being; that they can quickly rebalance from excesses by fasting for a day or taking some medicinal food or soup; that the natural way of healing the body is both possible and easy if we do not knock ourselves too far from center for too long. And most of all I want them to know that, mistakes and all, I did the best I knew at all times.

I remember vividly a deep heart-to-heart talk we had one day in the car, when Shana was about seven and Kaila four. "Why," they wanted to know, "don't we eat the same food that other people eat? It tastes good." I explained to them that I had done a lot of studying about food and that what I had learned was that food that tastes especially good is not always good for us. "I wish it wasn't so," I told them. "I wish I could eat chocolate every day and Hungarian sausage and potato salad with lots of mayonnaise, and French bread with butter and cheese on it. But I usually don't eat these things because although they taste good in my mouth, I don't like how I feel or how I look when I do eat them. So I have to make a choice and not take some things I like (like certain foods) in order to get others I like better (like being healthy and looking good)."

They listened intently. "But how about me?" Kaila asked. "Why can't I have real chocolate chip cookies and bologna sandwiches?" I took a long breath, to get more time to think. "Well," I finally said, "it's my job as a mother to take care of you and help you become a healthy, happy human being. I have to do my job the best I can. How can I give you food that I think is bad for you? If you grow up and eventually decide to eat your cookies and your bologna, it's your choice; if you get sick, it's also your problem. But now, if you get sick, it's my problem—I'm the one who has to stay up with you all night and put compresses on you and rub your feet. You can be sure that I'm going to do everything I can to keep you from getting sick. And that means that I won't buy you food that I think is bad for you."

There was no further comment, and I've never again had to explain myself.

Open Letter To Parents And Teachers

I want to bring to your attention an apparently small matter which is of great concern to me, and I'm sure that you'll see why once you have the facts.

Several times this school year our child has come home with no appetite for lunch. Every time it turned out that there had been candy, sweets, cupcakes, or similar "goodies" at school, either for a party of some kind or for no particular reason. A few times she came home with a bagful of candy.

It is an unfortunate fact that in our society the presence of sugared sweets is all-pervasive and children are taught very early that "candy is love." Worse, that sweets, ice cream, jams, jellies, sugar-coated sprinkles and cereals are not only good food, but that they are specifically children's food.

However, much medical research over the past two decades has linked sugar consumption with not only cavities and obesity but ulcers, heart disease, and behavioral problems. By displacing more nutritious food from the diet, sugar throws many of the body's functions off balance.

We discourage our child from eating sugar-sweetened foods. Although we have none at home and as a rule don't buy any, she does encounter them among her friends. There is not much we can do about this. However, when school becomes a candy store, I feel that as a concerned parent I must speak up. Banning sugar falls in the same category as banning liquor or cigarettes; perhaps desirable, but unenforceable. The next best thing is to become aware of the ill effects of sugar consumption so that those wishing to use it or give it to their children at least won't be under the delusion that it's "good" for them.

The Natural Lunch Box

BY BARBARA JACOBS

My son Jesse is six and loves to cook. Last week, as we were discussing his first days at school, I asked him what he would like to take in his lunchbox. We came up with many family favorites, plus a few new inspirations.

These recipes have been developed with children's lunches in mind, but they have many other possibilities. With a little imagination, by altering the proportions of the ingredients (or adding liquid—water or stock—if necessary), you can convert the sandwich fillings into tasty salad dressings, sauces for cooked vegetables or pasta, or party dips. Many of my guests, both children and adults, who have had little or no previous exposure to whole foods, enjoy them immensely. I hope you and your children and friends enjoy them as much as we do.

Note: For a smoother consistency, such as might be desired for a creamy sauce or salad dressing, you might want to use an electric blender. Otherwise, a Japanese suribachi is useful. The suribachi is a ceramic bowl (small, medium, or large) that has a grooved interior surface for grinding. It is also attractive enough to double as a serving dish.

Tofu Sandwich Filling

2 cakes tofu
5 pitted umeboshi plums
1 stalk celery, finely minced
½ small onion, minced (or a few scallions, minced)
3 tablespoons sesame butter or tahini
½ cucumber, finely chopped (optional)
½ cup olives, finely chopped (optional)

Boil tofu in enough water to cover for 5 minutes. Drain and let cool. Mash umeboshi to a paste. Add celery and onion, crushing the vegetables slightly. Add tofu and blend until mixture is spreadable. Add sesame butter and blend thoroughly. Add cucumber or olives, if desired.

Miso-Tahini Sandwich Filling
1 cup tahini
3 cups water or vegetable stock
½ cup minced onion (or scallion)
¼ cup grated zucchini or summer squash, or grated carrot, or diced cooked vegetables
2 tablespoons brown rice miso, diluted in 1 tablespoon water or vegetable stock
1 teaspoon fresh dill, cut very fine (optional)

Using a medium heat, "roast" tahini in a cast-iron frying pan, stirring constantly to prevent burning, until it bubbles and smells nutty. Reduce flame to as low as possible. Add the water (or stock) slowly, stirring until smooth. Then add the onion (or scallion) and vegetables of your choice. Stirring occasionally, cook until the vegetables are tender. Turn off heat. Add the miso and blend ingredients well. Add dill, if desired. Store in refrigerator.

Bean Spread

Any leftover cooked beans can be used for a delicious, hearty sandwich filling. Just purée and, for a more zesty flavor, add a little finely diced onion or scallion.

Rice Balls

Rice balls are a traditional Japanese food. They make a very satisfying lunch and are excellent food for traveling or picnics. If made properly, they will stay fresh for days. The saltiness of the pickled plum in the center acts as a preservative, and the nori seals in the rice.
1 handful cooked brown rice
1 sheet nori (seaweed), toasted
½ pitted umeboshi plum (or for children, ¼ plum)

Toast nori by passing both sides of the folded sheet over a medium flame until green. With wet hands, shape the rice into a flat patty, compressing the grains tightly. (Wet hands as necessary to prevent the grains from sticking.) When you have a smooth shape, make a hole in the center with your thumb and insert the umeboshi. Then plug up the hole with a little more rice.

Divide the toasted nori into quarters and, keeping hands moist to prevent the nori from sticking, use one of these pieces to cover one side of the rice patty. Turn the patty over and do the same to the other side. Patch up any uncovered spots with smaller pieces of nori. The nori should form a dry, smooth, tight black cover over the rice.

To pack rice balls for a lunchbox, wrap each one loosely in waxed paper. When made flat on the top and bottom, they stack very neatly and are easy to eat.

Grain-Vegetable Turnovers
MAKES SIX TURNOVERS
Dough:
> 2 cups whole wheat pastry flour
> ½ teaspoon sea salt
> ⅓ cup corn oil
> ½ cup water

Filling:
> ¼ cup each onion, celery, and carrot, minced (or ¾ cup leftover cooked vegetables)
> 2 tablespoons tamari

Glaze:
> 1 egg, beaten
> 1 tablespoon tamari or shoyu

Preheat oven to 350°. Combine the flour and salt. Add corn oil and mix lightly until flour and oil form little balls the size of peas. Add water and mix lightly; do not actually knead the dough. (It will be a little wet.) Set the dough aside and mix filling ingredients thoroughly. Dust rolling surface with 2-3 tablespoons flour. Make a ball of dough about 2 inches in diameter and roll out into a 6-inch circle. Put about ¼ cup of the filling on one half of the circle. Moisten the edges of the circle with a little water, then fold the other half of the dough over the filling. Press around the edge with a moistened fork and trim edges to ½ inch. Place the turnovers on a cookie sheet and brush the top with egg-tamari glaze. Bake for 1 hour.

Variation: For dessert turnovers, use your favorite pie filling. For a sweet glaze mix 1 egg with 2 tablespoons apple cider (or other fruit juice) or 1 tablespoon Yinnie rice syrup.

Coleslaw with Umeboshi Dressing
This salad can be a tangy accompaniment to Alphabet Soup.
> ½ medium head cabbage, grated
> ½ teaspoon sea salt
> water to cover
> 7 umeboshi plums
> ½ medium onion, diced
> ½ cup sesame or safflower oil
> ⅔ cup cold water
> 2 tablespoons parsley, finely chopped

Sprinkle cabbage lightly with salt. Toss well with hands, squeezing cabbage while mixing. Cover with water and let rest while preparing dressing. If a suribachi is used, first mash the plums, then add the diced onion, crushing it as you mix it in, and mix in oil until it is well blended with plums and onions; lastly, add the water and mix well. If a blender is used, first put in diced onion and umeboshi plums, then oil, and blend until smooth; add water little by little while blender is going, and stop when dressing is a uniform consistency. Drain the cabbage, squeezing it to remove excess liquid. Add salad dressing and toss lightly. Garnish with parsley.

Alphabet Soup
½ cup beets, cut into chunks
4 cups butternut squash, cut into chunks
7 cups water
1 tablespoon sesame oil
1 cup celery, diced
1 cup fresh corn kernels
2 cups green or wax beans, cut in 1-inch pieces
1 cup carrot, diced
1½ teaspoon sea salt
2 cups water
1 cup whole wheat alphabet noodles
1 cup water
1 medium leek, cut in ½ slices (separate greens and whites)

Pressure-cook the squash and beets in 4 cups water for 10 minutes. Place the pot under cold running water to reduce pressure; when pressure is down, purée the vegetables in a food mill or blender. In another pot heat oil slightly. Add the rest of the vegetables in the order given, and then the purée. Add the salt plus 2 cups water. Bring to a boil, reduce heat, and simmer for 45 minutes. Add alphabet noodles, the white part of the leek, and 1 cup water, and cook for 10 more minutes. Add leek greens and cook for 10 more minutes.

Wheat Gluten (Seitan)
Wheat gluten is not only an excellent source of vegetable-quality protein, it is also fun to make and is extremely versatile. The meat-like texture of the gluten enhances sandwiches, soups, grain casseroles, and vegetable stews. You can also enjoy it in the form of shish-kebabs and cutlets, and just about anything else you can think of! This recipe can be doubled or tripled. The unused gluten can be kept, refrigerated, up to 5 days. This recipe yields 2 cups uncooked gluten.
6 cups flour (unbleached white, whole wheat, or both)
4 cups lukewarm water

Place flour in a large mixing bowl. Add the water, mixing well, 1 cup at a time. Knead thoroughly, about 10 minutes, or until the dough forms a smooth ball. (This kneading is important: it activates the gluten in the flour.) Let the dough rest, uncovered, for about 10 minutes. Then fill the bowl with cold water and let the dough rest in the water for 10 minutes.

Begin to knead the dough in the water. When the water looks cloudy, drain it off and refill the bowl, this time with warm water. Repeat this process of kneading the dough and draining off the water, using warm and cold water alternately. As the dough is kneaded in the water, it will fall apart somewhat. Be careful not to lose any pieces of dough: sometimes a colander (not a strainer) is helpful in retaining all the pieces of dough. If whole wheat flour is used, the bran will also be washed away with the cloudy starch. As the water becomes clearer after repeated "washings" of the dough, the little pieces of gluten will begin to adhere to one another, and eventually they will form one large, soft, rubbery lump. The dough has been washed sufficiently when the water is clear. (Test by squeezing the gluten: The excess liquid should be almost clear.)

Gluten Steaks

There are many ways to cook the gluten once it is at this stage, but the simplest way to prepare it for use in sandwiches is to make "seitan," as follows:

2 cups uncooked gluten
water to just cover
¼ cup tamari (or to taste)
1 tablespoon grated fresh ginger
2 tablespoons sesame oil
3-inch strip kombu

Slice the gluten as for sandwiches. Put the cut gluten in a pot together with water to cover, tamari, ginger, and oil. Cut the kombu strip into very small pieces with a scissors and add. Bring to a boil, then reduce heat and cover. Simmer, checking periodically, until all the liquid is absorbed. This will take about 40 minutes to 1 hour. The long cooking is necessary for the pieces of gluten to completely absorb all the cooking liquid and its flavor. Instead of boiling, you can pressure-cook 20 minutes.

The seitan is done when it is a uniform color inside and out. If it is too salty, put the finished gluten in a bowl of cold water, which will draw out the excess tamari (which can be reserved for use in other dishes).

Carob Fudge

1 pound rice malt
2 cups peanut butter (preferably chunky)
¾ teaspoon sea salt
2 cups roasted carob powder
¼ cup water

½ cup roasted peanuts (optional)

Combine the syrup and peanut butter in a cast-iron frying pan (or double-boiler) over medium heat. (You may want to use a flame tamer under the pan to spread the heat evenly.) Stir until well blended, then add salt and carob, mixing well. Add water gradually, stirring constantly. Cook over a low flame for about 15 minutes, stirring occasionally. Turn out into a pie plate. Wet hands with cold water and smooth the top of the fudge. Refrigerate for 2 hours, or until set.

Apple-Lemon Kanten

Kanten, or agar, a sea vegetable, makes a light dessert that is similar to "Jello."

10 cups apple cider or juice
4 cups water (or more juice or cider)
⅛ teaspoon sea salt
7 tablespoons agar flakes
6 medium apples, cored and sliced
1 tablespoon grated lemon rind
juice of 1 medium lemon
¼ teaspoon cinnamon

Place cider (or juice) and water in a saucepan and, while they are heating, prepare other ingredients. When the cider and water come to a boil, reduce heat, and add salt and agar. Simmer for 5 minutes, stirring constantly. Stir in apples, lemon rind, lemon juice, and cinnamon. Simmer for 15 minutes more, pour in dish, and chill until set.

Oat-Raisin Cookies
APPROXIMATELY 30 COOKIES

3 cups rolled oats
1 cup raisins
1½ cups apple cider (or juice)
⅔ cup corn oil
2½ cups whole wheat pastry flour
¼—½ teaspoon sea salt
1 cup roasted sunflower seeds

Preheat oven to 350°F. Dry-roast oats in a cast-iron frying pan over medium heat, stirring constantly to prevent burning, until they smell nutty. Meanwhile, simmer the raisins in juice for 5 minutes. Place the hot oats in a mixing bowl and add the oil immediately, tossing lightly to coat. Drain raisins (reserving liquid), and add. Add pastry flour, salt, and seeds, and toss lightly. Add the raisin liquid and mix well. Drop teaspoonfuls onto an oiled cookie sheet and pat slightly on top, flattening to about ½ thick. Bake for 45 minutes.

Cooking for Mommy and Daddy

BY KATHLEEN BELLICCHI

T he first thing I ever cooked all by myself, besides cake mixes and scrambled eggs, was vegetable soup. One afternoon I found myself home alone—a rare occurrence in itself since I had three brothers and two sisters at the time—and had the urge to make the house my own in the same way my mother did: by cooking. What could be better than a pot of soup simmering on the stove, thick and creamy, with big, juicy chunks of vegetables, making the whole kitchen smell wonderful? I began by getting out a heavy pot. It seemed like the best pot to use to make the soup I had in mind; a heavy pot is ideal for thick soup because it holds heat well, allowing the soup to cook down and become creamy over a low flame.

After choosing my pot, I looked in the refrigerator and took out all the vegetables that looked good to me. I cut only the ones that didn't fit in the pot. I don't remember exactly what I used, but it was probably a carrot, a stalk of celery, a few small onions and, happily, some mushrooms. I added water until it seemed there was enough for a soup and then began looking around for something to make it creamy, as well as to make it unusual and uniquely mine. I found a box of barley and used a handful to thicken the soup; then I looked through herbs and spices. Seasonings were very foreign to me, so much so that they scared me; but after carefully smelling each jar, I decided on a bay leaf (I had seen my mother use it in stews) and, throwing caution to the wind, I put in some basil.

I had some idea of how much salt to use from my experience making scrambled eggs; so I put about half a teaspoon in the pot; then I put the pot on the stove. I turned on the flame and watched as it began to cook—it seemed to take so long. I remember I ate most of it before it was really cooked—the carrots were still a little crispy and the barley chewy, but I thought it was perfect. The idea of putting ingredients in a pot, adding water, and using fire to create something that smelled and tasted good was magical and exciting to me.

I also cooked dinner for my family one night when I was working on a Girl Scout badge. The rules stated that I had to have my mother work with me, and it wasn't nearly as much fun as making a pot of soup by myself. I enjoyed helping my mother when she was cooking for holidays or parties, but best of all I liked making choices and decisions by myself when I cooked.

I also learned at an early age what it means to have too many cooks in the kitchen when my brother, my sisters, and I made brunch one Sunday morning. We completed our meal, but chaos reigned throughout. After that, when we had the urge to cook together, we worked in pairs. I especially liked cooking with my older brother Michael because he was much more adventurous in his choice of ingredients than I was.

I had one cookbook then that I liked very much. It was written for young people and was very thorough in explaining every detail of preparation. When I used my cookbook, it was like having a friend in the kitchen to help me out.

The following is a simple meal, complete with dessert, that children can cook for their parents. It will amply serve four people.

Vegetable Soup
Rice
Broccoli
Oatmeal cookies
Tea

When you plan to cook, check the refrigerator and pantry early in the day to see if you have all the ingredients you will need. It would also be helpful to have a timer so you don't get involved in a project and forget something else. Read over the instructions for the meal beforehand so you will have an idea of the meal as a whole. To cook this meal you will need:

2 cups short grain brown rice
1 large carrot
2 stalks celery
1 large onion (or 4 small ones)
¼ cup barley
1 bay leaf
1 teaspoon basil
1 cup whole wheat pastry flour
2 cups rolled oats
½ cup raisins
1/3 cup corn oil
¼ cup maple syrup
¼ teaspoon cinnamon

1 bunch broccoli
oil for sautéeing
shoyu
sea salt
lemon
parsley—1 sprig
bancha tea

Before you begin, wash any dishes in the sink and tidy up the kitchen. While cooking the meal, wash utensils as you go along—everything seems to flow better when you keep your space neat and orderly; it also saves you from washing a sinkful of things when you are done.

After planning a meal, I think about the dishes I will be preparing and how long it will take for each one to cook; then I plan the order of cooking so everything will be ready to serve at the same time. For this meal I will begin by putting on the rice, then the soup, and then preparing the cookies and putting them in the oven. While the cookies are baking, I'll cut and cook the broccoli; then I'll put on the tea just before it's time to eat.

It will probably take about two hours to cook this meal, so start early enough. You don't want to feel pressured when your family or friends peer into the kitchen asking how long until dinner is ready.

Before you begin preparing each dish, read over the recipe and gather all the ingredients and utensils you will need.

Rice
   2 cups short grain brown rice
   4 cups water
   $1/8$ teaspoon sea salt

Utensils:
   1 medium-size heavy pot
   1 wire-mesh strainer
   1 measuring cup
   $1/8$ teaspoon measuring spoon
   flame tamer

Measure 2 cups of rice and put it in the cooking pot. Wash the rice by adding water to cover and mixing with your hands; you will see dust particles and rice husks floating to the top. Pour off the water, placing the strainer underneath to catch the rice. Now add 4 cups of clean water to the rice, together with $1/8$ teaspoon salt, and put it on the stove. Cover the pot, turn the heat on high, and bring the rice to a boil (it will take approximately 10 minutes). Turn the timer to 10 minutes so you will not forget to check it. After it boils, turn the heat down low and put a metal flame tamer under the pot. This will distribute the heat evenly and prevent the rice from sticking to the bottom of the pot. Set the timer on 45 minutes after you turn the flame down, and go on to make the soup. When the bell on the timer rings, take the rice off the stove, put it on the table with a mat underneath (so you don't scorch the table), and take the cover off. Fluff the rice gently, mixing from bottom to top, and cover with a bamboo sushi mat.

Vegetable Barley Soup
  1 large carrot
  2 stalks celery
  1 large onion (or 4 small ones)
  oil to brush the cooking pot for sautéeing
  5 cups water
  ½ teaspoon sea salt
  ¼ cup barley
  1 bay leaf
  ¼ teaspoon basil
  2 teaspoons shoyu

Utensils:
  vegetable brush
  cutting board
  knife
  soup pot
  wooden spoon
  measuring spoons—½ teaspoon, ¼ teaspoon, teaspoon
  You may not think these are the most exciting vegetables, but they are easy to cut and they look and taste good together.
  Wash the carrot and celery to remove any clinging dirt. Place the cutting board on the counter or table you plan to use. If the regular cutting surface in the kitchen is too high for you, choose a lower surface. When standing, the ideal height for cutting is about 2 inches above the top of your legs. Use a vegetable cutting knife with a blade 5 to 7 inches long.
  It is as easy to use a large knife as it is to use a small paring knife and, for cutting a number of vegetables, it is quicker. If you are right-handed, hold the knife in your right hand (reverse directions if you are left-handed). Hold the vegetables with your left hand, fingers together, with the fingernails pressed against the back of the knife. This makes it easy to cut evenly, and it is impossible to cut yourself. Cut each stalk of celery into four equal pieces. Place the soup pot on the stove, turn the heat to medium, and brush the bottom of the pot

lightly with oil. Put the onions in the pot and stir them with a wooden spoon. After 3 minutes add the celery and then the carrots. Stir the vegetables for a minute and then add 5 cups water, ½ teaspoon salt, ¼ cup barley, a bay leaf, and a pinch of basil. When the soup boils, cover the pot. Turn the flame down a little, and let it simmer (simmer means a very low boil—the soup is bubbling slowly) until you are ready to serve dinner. Check the soup from time to time. If it is boiling or looks as though the liquid is evaporating, turn the flame down. After the soup has been cooking 30 minutes, add 2 teaspoons shoyu (tamari soy sauce), let it cook for a few minutes, and then take a taste. Take out the bay leaf. Add a bit more shoyu if you think it is needed.

Before you go on to the cookies look at the rice and see if it is cooking properly. Is the water being absorbed by the rice? If not, turn up the flame a bit. Is the rice sticking to the bottom of the pot? If it is, turn the flame down slightly. Check on the soup also.

Oatmeal Cookies
   1 cup whole wheat pastry flour
   2 cups rolled oats
   ½ cup raisins
   ¼ cup corn oil
   ¹/₃ cup maple syrup
   ¼ teaspoon sea salt
   ¼ teaspoon cinnamon
   ½ cup water

Utensils:
   1 mixing bowl
   wooden spoon
   measuring cup
   soup spoon
   cookie sheet (2 if you have them)
   metal spatula
   cooling rack
   measuring spoons—¼ teaspoon, ½ teaspoon

Turn on the oven to 350°F. If you need to strike a match to light the oven, ask for help if you have never done it before. Put the oven rack in the middle of the oven to bake the cookies. Measure out 1 cup whole wheat pastry flour, 2 cups rolled oats, ½ cup raisins, ¼ teaspoon salt, ¼ teaspoon cinnamon, and place them in the mixing bowl. With the wooden spoon, mix everything together. Measure out ¼ cup corn oil, add it to the dry ingredients, and mix with the spoon until the oil coats all the ingredients evenly. Add ¹/₃ cup maple syrup, mix it in, then stir in ½ cup water.

Brush the cookie sheet lightly with oil, and use a soup spoon to drop the cookies onto the sheet. Pick up a heaping spoonful of batter and drop it onto the sheet. Spread the batter out a little with the back side of the spoon to even out the shape of the cookie. They should be about 2 inches across. Put the cookies on the middle rack in the oven, and set the rest of the batter aside for a second batch. If you have another cookie sheet and room in the oven on the center rack, you can bake them all at once. Set the time for 15 minutes. When the bell rings, check the cookies. They are done when they have browned slightly on the bottoms and sides. Of course, the best test is to taste one!

Use the spatula to put the cookies on the cooling rack, then put your second batch in the oven. You will have approximately 15 to 18 cookies. The cooling rack allows the cookies to cool quickly and makes them crispy.

When the cookies are in the oven, you can wash and cut the broccoli for steaming. Steaming is the process of cooking food on a rack or in a basket placed over boiling water but not touching the water.

Broccoli
1 bunch broccoli
water for steaming

Utensils:
1 cutting board
knife
steamer, or pot with steaming basket

Wash each stalk of broccoli and shake out the excess water. Lay the stalks on the cutting board one at a time, and slice across with your knife about 3 inches below the floweret. Remember to keep your fingers together and your fingernails against the back of the knife. Hold the broccoli upside down so the floweret is resting on the cutting board, then cut through the stalk to separate the broccoli into bite-size pieces. Put 2 inches of water in the steaming pot, place the basket on or inside the pot depending on the type of steamer you are using, and turn the heat on high. When the water boils, put the broccoli in the steamer, put the cover on, and let it steam 8 minutes.

Take one piece out and taste it. I like it best when it is still bright green in color and the stalk is tender. Steaming baskets have a metal hook that lifts the basket out of the pot. If you don't have one of these, or if you would rather not use it, take the broccoli out of the steamer with a serving spoon. To season the broccoli, sprinkle on 1 teaspoon shoyu, if you wish.

Your dinner is cooked; it's time to set the table and serve the food. The presentation of a meal is as important and as much fun as the cooking itself. Choose bowls to complement the food and use contrasting colored vegetables, fruits, or flowers as a centerpiece.

Take the rice out of the cooking pot with a wooden spoon or rice paddle and put it in a bowl. A plain wooden bowl that is not shiny or lacquered on the inside is the best choice for rice. Place a small piece of parsley on top of the rice in the center of the bowl as a garnish. Arrange the broccoli in a serving bowl and garnish it with a few slices of lemon. To serve the soup, put a piece of onion in each bowl, 2 slices each of carrot and celery, and some of the barley and broth. Put the cookies on a plate or in a basket to serve along with the tea after dinner. And now call everyone—it's time to eat!

Kids in the Kitchen

BY REBECCA THEURER WOOD

Mid-summer means the children are around the house more than during the school year. It's a relaxing time for them but sometimes relaxation can turn to boredom and you need to use your wits to help them keep busy. One sure-fire winner is cooking.

Kids can do more in the kitchen than set the table and wash the dishes. My four-year-old loves cutting vegetables, my six-year-old is into stirring, and many a time my ten-year-old prepares a whole meal. They're all adept at making menageries with bread dough, decorating cakes with slivered almonds, and they've tested the recipes that follow. The only ground rule is—no commotion in the kitchen. And, generally, they don't "commote" because cooking is so much fun.

Macaroni Salad
SERVES 4

   4 cups cooked macaroni shells or bows
   1 cup peas
   1 cup broccoli flowerets
   ½ cup carrots, cut into rounds

Have the children shuck the peas while you steam the broccoli and carrots lightly and make the salad dressing. Lightly steam peas. Allow vegetables to cool and toss with pasta and your favorite dressing, or use the one below.

Tahini Salad Dressing
YIELDS ½ CUP

   ¼ cup tahini
   juice of one lemon
   ¼ cup water
   1 teaspoon umeboshi paste, or 1 whole plum, mashed

Combine tahini and lemon juice in a small bowl and mix well. Add water slowly and blend until creamy. Mix in umeboshi.

Sweet Carrot Butter
YIELDS 2 CUPS

3 cups carrot chunks
¼ cup water
pinch sea salt
¼ cup tahini

Place carrots, water, and salt in a pressure cooker, bring to pressure, and cook for 5 minutes; or pot cook with a little more water, tightly covered, for 15-20 minutes or until soft. Place tahini in small skillet and roast until just golden. Run carrots through food mill and stir in tahini. Spread on crepes, toast, or pancakes.

If your children are uncomfortable with vegetable desserts, find the right enticing name and they'll ask for seconds.

Buckwheat Crepes
8 LARGE CREPES

2 cups buckwheat flour
¼ cup whole wheat pastry flour
¼ teaspoon sea salt
4 cups water

Mix ingredients together and allow to rest for 45 minutes. Heat crepe pan (4 inch high sides) or small skillet until a drop of water sizzles on it. A well seasoned skillet requires oiling for just the first crepe; however, if they stick lightly oil the pan for each crepe. Pour batter into a large measuring cup or pitcher. Pour batter onto skillet, lift skillet and rotate to spread the batter in a thin layer. Cook over medium flame for 3-4 minutes, turn and cook for 2 more minutes. Top with maple syrup, fruit butter, squash purée, fish sauce, or creamy vegetable dishes. Crepes are delicious for breakfast, lunch, or dinner. They also make fine lunch-box fare.

Strawberry Sauce
YIELDS 2¼ CUPS

1 cup water
¼ cup maple syrup
pinch sea salt
1 tablespoon kuzu dissolved in 2 tablespoons water
1 pint strawberries, sliced thin

Place water, syrup, and salt in saucepan and bring to boil. Stir in kuzu and simmer for 2 minutes, mixing continuously. Pour hot kuzu mixture over strawberries. Place several tablespoons of strawberry filling on each crepe, roll up, and serve hot.

Children enjoy washing, hulling, and slicing strawberries. If there's going to be a lot of tasting you might want to start with extra berries.

Corn-On-The-Cob
This is my favorite way to prepare fresh corn.

Let the children husk the corn. Put them out on the lawn with one bag for the corn and another for the husks. Even the youngest children enjoy this summer ritual.

Place husks on the bottom of a large pressure cooker or pot with a cover. Add corn, ½ cup water, and a pinch of sea salt. Pressure cook for 3 minutes if the corn was just picked, up to 5 minutes if less fresh. (Pot cook for 6-10 minutes.)

Place cooker under a small stream of cold water to quickly release pressure. Serve corn with umeboshi—each person rubs their corn lightly with a bit of whole plum or spreads a bit of paste on with a knife. Umeboshi tastes just like butter and salt on corn!

Corn-cob Soup Stock
For an unusually sweet and nutritious stock, remove husks from the pot, add all the empty cobs, a piece of kombu, and water to cover. Simmer for 30 minutes or so, strain out cobs and kombu, and proceed with your soup.

Amesake
YIELDS 2½ QUARTS

Children love amesake, and a more wholesome food is hard to imagine. Simply fermented grain, it's sweet, easy to digest, and full of enzymes and bacteria that augment our own intestinal flora and assist in the digestion of other foods. I make up a big batch that can keep in the refrigerator for two weeks (if it doesn't get eaten up sooner). Most grains, in conjunction with sweet rice, can be turned into amesake. Here's one of my children's favorites.

2 cups millet
4 cups sweet rice
14 cups water
4 cups koji rice

Wash and soak millet and sweet rice overnight. In the morning pressure cook for 25 minutes or pot cook for 30 minutes. Place in a large ceramic bowl and let cool just till you can put a finger down into it without saying, "Ouch." Mix koji in well, cover with a damp towel and let it sit in a warm place for 10 to 14 hours or until it has a sweet-but-not sour fragrance. (An oven with a pilot light works well.)

When incubation is complete, remove amesake to a pot and simmer over a medium flame for a few minutes. Stir frequently and use a flame distributor to prevent scorching. Cool and refrigerate. Serve as pudding and let your children "doctor" it as they like with fruits, nuts, carob powder, spices, etc. Use amesake and your (their) imagination to create an endless variety of healthful sweet treats.

One of my children's favorite summertime amesake treats is to purée it, and turn it into "ice cream" in the freezer. To produce a creamy consistency, use an ice cream churner if you have one. Simply follow churning directions.

Fruit Salad

On a hot day when your children have "nothing to do" ask them to make a fruit salad. My kids lose themselves in cutting the fruit into different shapes, combining, tasting, and finally, serving their masterpiece. If you need to help you might scoop out orange shells to make individual serving bowls, or toast nuts or seeds to add. Shredded coconut or a sprig of fresh mint makes an attractive garnish.

Here's one example of a fruit salad combination. This one yields about 4 cups.

½ cantaloupe
1 thick slice water melon
1 pint blueberries
1 cup cherries
juice of one-half lemon or orange

Cut melons into chunks. Add berries and cherries and squeeze citrus juice over. Toss and serve.

Apple Kanten
YIELDS APPROXIMATELY 3 CUPS

My children make this "jello" frequently. It's quick and is an acceptable dessert they can make all by themselves. It is soothing to the digestive system and medicinal to the lungs, which makes me happy. Fresh fruit may be added. However, then it becomes only dessert, rather than dessert and medicine.

1 bar kanten (or 2 tablespoons agar flakes, or 1 teaspoon agar powder)
3 cups apple juice
pinch sea salt
2 tablespoons kuzu
¼ cup cold water

Rinse kanten (if using bar) under cold water ad squeeze dry. Place apple juice and salt into a pot and break kanten into it. Bring to a boil and stir and simmer until kanten is completely dissolved. Dissolve kuzu in cold water and stir into juice mixture. Stir continuously until it turns clear. Rinse a bowl with cold water and pour hot juice mixture into it and allow to set.

The Ultimate Almond Cookie
YIELDS 1½ DOZEN
3 cups almonds
¼-½ cup apple juice
juice of 1 orange
1 teaspoon vanilla
½ teaspoon cinnamon
1 cup yinnie syrup or barley malt
½ teaspoon sea salt

Grind almonds in a blender, a few at a time, to make a meal. Add enough apple juice to make a smooth paste. Combine almond paste with remaining ingredients. Drop onto a well oiled baking sheet. Press lightly with a fork. Bake on a high rack in a preheated oven at 325° F. for 10 minutes or just until they are golden. Watch closely—this cookie may burn quickly.

Education

Interview: Shlomo and Nela Carlebach

BY JOB MATUSOW

EWJ: *This issue of East West Journal is about children and play. I'm sitting here looking at your child. You're a holy man; how does it feel to be her father?*
Carlebach: I wish I would be a holy man! Anyway, the closest I've ever gotten to the coming of the Messiah is when my baby was born.

Suddenly someone told me, "there is a woman calling you outside the synagogue." Right away I knew my wife was sending someone to let me know that I had to come home fast. I want you to know that I was so high at this moment, I thought, I'll never do another thing wrong again in my whole life. It really is true.

Talking about babies, I think that the world makes one mistake. The world says, "Children are playing and adults are real." The saddest thing is that it's the other way around: children, they are real. The older we get, the more we play around. The saddest thing is there is no peace in the world. "Let them go to war, let them kill each other," we say. We adults sitting here, we say we are the real people. We are safe. But if they would know that they are fooling around and the children are the real people, they would be a little more careful about that which is most real.

I was learning yesterday something very deep: the greatest evil in the world is not what you do wrong. The greatest evil in the world is if what you do, you don't do wholeheartedly. If you do it, do it completely, do it totally. I see a poor man on the street and I give him a dime. Why don't I give it to him completely?

EWJ: *What do you mean by completely? Do you mean you should give him a dollar?*
Carlebach: No, I mean if I only have a dime, the one dime I give out, I just give him from the outside of my heart. Why didn't I put the inside of my heart into it? And then if I put the inside of my heart into it, I discover that the inside of my heart has another inside.

In the Zoharhakodash (that's a textbook of Jewish mysticism), it says, "The outside of a higher world becomes the inside for the lower world and the outside of this world becomes the inside of a lower world again." That means for somebody in a higher world, his outside for a person in a lower level is already called inside. Let's say, for instance, this is my inside today and if maybe tomorrow I would reach a higher world, I would realize this was still outside, and I was not inside yet.

Until children learn how to speak, to form words, everything is complete. The only sad thing is the moment they speak. Since words, in a very strange way, are coming from a very high world. God created the world with words, with ten words. But since it's such a delicate thing, you can lie with words.

EWJ: *Do you believe that words may be obsolete as we develop the ability to communicate psychically-telepathically?*
Carlebach: No, I'll tell you, there are two levels of words. One level of words is for information. Then on a higher level of words, I need the words not because I didn't know it but because it is so deep when you say it. For example, when I say to my wife "I love you," it's not because she didn't know it. It's not information. It's a much deeper word because I didn't know before and I say, "Oh! Thank you God. It's really beautiful news to me." Hah! We knew it before or I wouldn't be standing on Mount Sinai. The beautiful thing is that He said it. That level of words is the real level of words, whole words. . . deep words. . . .

Well, ask me something strong, brother.

EWJ: *You say you still have to use the words. I say no, that when I look in your eyes and you look in my eyes and I know I love you and you love me, you don't need the words.*
Carlebach: God created words for a purpose; words themselves are beautiful. If you remember someone told you, "I love you," it's a very whole thing. The words themselves are not on the level of information. It's on the level they have been said.

The world always thinks prayer means to let God know what I need. So they ask, "Doesn't God know before?" But the words of prayer are not words to tell God what I need; He knows before. But the words when I utter them become vessels to what I need, if I say them before God.
Nela: There are so many different kinds of words. There are holy words and there are words which are very unholy. If I say to my baby, "Listen, you better go ahead and be strong and be beautiful and grow with life, and I want you to be a nurse," right away I'm putting my baby in a mold with my words. If my words are holy words and I say to my baby, "Please be who you are in the utmost of the utmost ways and whatever you have now as a baby, please hold onto it," then my baby has a place to grow.

My words can cut her off; my words can make her grow. When she grows, she can learn how to utter words that will give her strength and growth or she can utter words that will cut other people down around her.

The biggest disappointment children have now is because their parents say, "I want you to do this" and they look at their parents and the words don't match. People have to learn how to educate their child mostly by saying what they really are. As Shlomo said, the worst evil is not being evil, but rather not being completely good. If I have one thing I stand for, and I'm a terrible woman in every other way, but I have that one thing, and my baby sees that one thing is real, she will learn more from that one thing in its utmost, from its word, from its expression, from everything, than from the totality of my lies.

When I talk to my child, if I say to her "I really love you; go to sleep and stop making so much noise," the love gets lost in the command, in the wish. But if I love her without conditions and then later on I say, "Please go to sleep," that's something else. Nowadays we love, and we bribe. I know so many women who woo their babies: "I love you, baby, but have a cookie and be quiet." So words can be holy, but they are debased. Shlomo gave a Torah lesson once and said anything that is really holy and true and beautiful is also the most corrupt. There is nothing more beautiful than a man and a woman together, and that is taken and brought so low, so down. There is nothing more beautiful than money. It's a holy thing from God, but we've taken. . . .

EWJ: *Money? I don't agree.*

Carlebach: No, money itself comes from a very high place, only people don't know what to do with it. Reb Nachmun says the two most misused things in the world are sex and money. Because they come from such a high place, if you don't know what to do with them, it's absolutely degrading and it rolls down. Money is a very high thing. If I have money in my pocket, I can do the greatest things in the world with it. I can build the Holy Temple with it. God put something in the world. There is such a thing. God put it there, and we have free choice what to do with it. But since it comes from such a high place, the choice is so strong. I want you to know something very deep, I was learning with my kids. Anything which is good and sweet but is compromised may be good, but that thing which is completely uncompromised is called holy. The moment you start compromising, it's not holy any more. Money comes from such a high place; it's holy, but if you compromise a little bit here, a little bit there, it's already not holy. Holy means uncompromised.

Learning from Children
You Don't Have To Be a Parent To Love Kids

BY BILL BURNS

"**B**illburns, Billburns. . . ." For four-year-old Jesse my name had become a mantra, and his chanting always brought results in the form of immediate attention. But this time he was treading on thin ice. Two stories past his bedtime he was still very much awake, so I told him he could wait up for his parents if he stayed in bed and stopped talking. I figured the quiet activity of reading (looking at the pictures and remembering the accompanying words) would lull him to sleep. Quiet for a while, then, "Billburns." I opened the door but before I could remind him of our deal he stopped me with a beautiful, clear smile and said, "I love you, Billburns."

I can think of few activities as satisfying and rewarding as spending time with children. But for me that feeling has only developed in the last two years. As a thirty-one-year-old single man, I had spent very little time with children since my own childhood. And my few experiences with them had generally been more grating than encouraging. For example, three years ago I rented a room from a couple with four children ranging in age from six months to six years. When I *could* get in the bathroom there was usually a diaper in the sink. Dinners were bouts of sibling squabbles and parental shushes. And several mornings a week I was awakened prematurely by heart-piercing crying. In search of peace and quiet I kept my distance. Besides, what could I talk about with a first-grader, or how could I entertain a two-year-old? I could probably remember how to play Duck Duck Goose, but don't ask me to recite Mother Goose. Only later when I got to know ten-year-old Alden did I realize that I had been seeing the circumstances, not the children.

Alden's mother Alexandra and I met each other through a Christian community but we'd spent little time together. One day after choir practice, a small group of us went out to lunch, and I found myself in the back of a station wagon with Alden. Small talk soon turned into a discussion of her feelings about her father's second marriage. I was impressed with her clarity of perception and the ease with which she spoke about a subject that could have been emotional dynamite. And I was enjoying myself.

At lunch we continued talking as she positioned herself between her mother and me. Then when the talk at the table turned to relationships, Alden said she thought Alexandra should marry me. Thick silence. Such audacity!

We hardly know each other. Pause. Let's see. Could she be onto something? Well, not a marriage, but the door was now open for a beautiful relationship with Alexandra. And by accepting Alden as an interesting and whole person I was on my way to seeing all children as sources of inspiration. Instead of being anxious about these swarms of dissidents whose main objective seemed to be to overthrow my peace of mind, I became excited about the fullness of their energies, their curiosities, and their potential to be my teachers.

Being willing to love a child is the most important qualification you need. If you can give a child your undivided attention, really listen to what he or she is saying or not saying, you are offering an invaluable gift. Patience helps. Sometimes a first meeting seems like a complete failure. Sylvie wouldn't even say hello to me the first time we met. I'm sure she left fingernail marks in her mother's thighs trying to hide from me. Then I visited her a few times at her home. There she was comfortable enough with her surroundings to open up. After a few games of hide and seek we were fast friends, and now she makes drawings for me and pesters her mother at least once a week to ask me over for dinner.

As soon as I start thinking I'm Mr. Wonderful with kids, though, my balloon springs a leak. Recently, one-year-old Rosie cried and clung to her mother everytime I came near her. I had been her Saturday morning babysitter practically since birth so this was unusual behavior from my small friend who used to smile and hold her arms out when she saw me. Her mother then realized that I was only around when Mom and Dad went out, so Rosie was equating my coming with her parents' leaving. I saw the strength and beauty of family ties and my need to support and join them in spirit instead of thinking of myself as a parental substitute.

Kids love to push to see what they can get away with, and in doing so they help you face up to your own thoughts and feelings with honesty. Try lying or backing down on a promise to a six-year-old. See if he or she doesn't call you on it and quote something you've forgotten you said six months ago. Last fall I was sitting in the lobby of a local Waldorf school thumbing through a book about pantomime when a first-grader asked me if I could do mime. I said I could, so he said, "Why don't you do some for us?" No harm in asking, right? I could have turned him down, but then I would have missed a nice workout and further insight into what makes a six-year-old laugh. Whenever my friend Suzin is in a bad mood, she seeks out her friends' children so she no longer has the luxury of doting on herself. After making someone else the focus of her attention, her mood always improves.

If you're interested in spending more time with children but worried about your lack of experience, start with a child you are attracted to who also likes you. Save the "problem child" for later. The advantage we have over parents is that we can choose the child we want to spend time with and we can come and go as we please. As in any relationship, however, trust takes time to develop, and the stronger the commitment the greater the rewards. As long as you are conscientious, don't worry about mistakes. I don't know a parent who doesn't think he or she completely blew it at one time or another. And you certainly don't need to be an expert on children's games. All you need is willingness to play. Children will barrage you with ideas and pull you into playrooms or backyards to the point where the problem is no longer where to start but how to stop.

Your stepping out and taking a chance can also help another group: single parents. By working outside the home to pay for food, rent, and clothing, they are pulled away from the very home they are trying to create and, more importantly, from the child they are creating it for. They need a break. Our Christian community set up a program to aid single mothers. Roughly based on the nationwide Big Brother program, our set-up asked the adult for a once-a-week-for-a-year commitment to one child. Unlike the Big Brother program, adults could be paired with children of the opposite sex depending on what the parent felt to be the need in each child's case. These growing relationships have given everyone involved a sense of love and extended family through community cooperation.

In opening up to children, I have tasted the pure joy of a baby, the refreshing curiosity of a toddler, and the audacity of a young adult—priceless training for a future father.

P.S. Jesse, I love you too.

Learning at Home

BY CATHY CREIGHTON

Cathy Creighton took her daughter, Eliza, out of school after the fifth grade. She writes of trying to "teach" Eliza at home and of Eliza's eventual development of her own learning methods.

It is rare to hear of a child who does not attend school. Yet it is not unheard of now, and it is becoming more acceptable. What is unusual about my fourteen-year-old daughter, Eliza, is that she has no overt substitute in her life for school education. She does not have a correspondence course, nor do my husband and I give her classes. No one expects her to learn anything taught in schools, nor has she had any conventional teachers since we began keeping her home after the fifth grade.

Eliza didn't drop out of school. She had always enjoyed school and done well. My husband and I kept her home because we were increasingly at odds with the results of sending her to school. Our family's attention and activity differed from the school's. The school sought to stimulate and broaden the child's mind; we sought to calm and channel. As our foci differed, our problems differed, and as our problems differed our solutions diverged.

Not knowing what would work, we at least wanted to stop doing what we knew didn't work. It became more interesting to watch our own failures than the failures of the prescribed education. We took the point of view that we, rather than the school teachers, were her caretakers and educators. We launched upon innumerable alternative methods, including correspondence courses, home study schedules of various subjects, and practical applications. As educators, we paid close attention to the results on Eliza and the rest of the family. Our failures became subtly fascinating as our focus broadened. We noticed that each idea we came up with on how to guide her resulted in adverse-side effects, emphasizing some aspect of Eliza or the family out of proportion to the rest. This created an endless series of problems, like weeding a garden. When you weed, you create an insect problem. When you spray, you create a soil problem. When you fertilize, you create a pollution problem. When you don't weed, strength emerges. When you don't spray, health emerges. And when you stop fertilizing, vital nourishment emerges. Only the basics can balance a natural garden successfully—soil, seed, sun, watchfulness, and time.

Similarly, in educating, when you give classes, you create worry. When you entertain, you distract. When you apply pressure, you incite rebellion. . . ad infinitum. We tired of our own efforts to educate Eliza—our participation slackened. As we overtly did less and less—verging on nothing at all—a very balanced and satisfying form of education began to emerge. We found that when you forego classes, you foster curiosity. When you stop entertaining, attention grows. When you release pressure, participation swells. We found that only the basics balance a natural education successfully—home, food, family and, of course, watchfulness and time.

Once the patterns of school and subject matter faded out in Eliza and in us, experience taught her. Younger brothers and sisters, her friends, the friends she thought she had, the food she eats, daily housekeeping, talking with her parents. . . even the mirror in the bathroom, the kitchen clock, and the calendar on the wall—all these and more give her special private classes every day. These are her teachers.

These teachers are as demanding as she allows them to be. She alone determines their strictness by varying the focus of her attention. Sometimes her attention is concentrated, and sometimes it isn't. Her homework is to watch, listen, express, observe, participate, reflect, and relax. It's easy for her because, without school patterns or educational images, that's what she does anyway.

Yesterday Eliza was cleaning the bathroom. David, aged three, decided to help, and I heard loud objections from Eliza, since David was doing more dirtying than dusting. He put scouring powder where she had already scrubbed and rinsed, and his dirty feet muddied the wet-mopped floor. For a while I heard nothing, then pleasant sounds of conversation and mild instruction. She had changed her approach mid-stream. She gave him the bathroom scale to do by himself, showed him how to apply just a little scouring powder and how to squeeze out the sponge so that it wouldn't drip while scrubbing. She had also washed his feet. With David, she was learning what a cheerful solution it is to find the source of a problem in our own attitude rather than in someone else's.

Eliza had studied ballet from the age of four. By the time she decided she wanted to end these classes seven years later, she had earned a full scholarship to the Cambridge School of Ballet, attended long sessions four days a week, and was very good. One evening, my husband and I returned from a late movie and found this note.

Dear Mom and Dad,

It's 7:30 and we're going to bed. The kids are happy and Mary ate well.

I was looking at my face in the mirror tonight for a long time. It's so different than it used to be! It used to be slender, delicate, emotional—a ballerina's face. It's hard for me to imagine wanting to be a ballerina now. Ballet was a tragic career to have chosen for myself. The dramatic, bittersweet ballerina image—that was my face before. Now I want to be peaceful, healthy— nothing special—just happy. Now my face is broader and stronger and clearer. Different.

We can talk about it in the morning. How was the movie? I hope you had a good time.

Lots of love,
Eliza Jane

Eliza was learning that her appetite for life is reflected in her own image.

To be continuously learning is not difficult for her, but natural. A truly difficult challenge would be to keep her from learning.

From younger brothers and sisters, Eliza learns child-care, patience, kindness, and love. From friends she learns about relationships. From food, she learns about her natural human needs. From housekeeping, she learns about activity. From conversation, she learns to speak accurately and listen carefully. She sees changes in the mirror, and from clock and calendar learns the rhythms of day and year. Her subject matter is simple and obvious yet subtle and substantial. Her education is as basic as common sense. Indeed, it is the understanding, the deepening, and the appreciation of common sense which turns common sense into infinite wonder.

The whole family benefits from this natural education. Home life is tremendously enhanced as each member becomes happier. Eliza's lessons from daily life relax her, affecting those older and younger. She becomes our teacher also. We learn that any individual is free to discover more than all the knowledge of civilization and humanity. So much we thought we had to do is neither necessary nor beneficial. Indeed the family is vitalized and strengthened by the presence of one relaxed teenager. The home grows more peaceful as her learning deepens.

Over the years we've had several visits from truant officers. For the most part they simply want to know that there is no child abuse involved, and sometimes they want to know why we're breaking the law. The last visit was a year ago. A pleasant, quiet-spoken young woman appeared on our doorstep one morning. We discussed the paradoxes of education. From the school's point of view—especially from the administration's point of view—society's expectations of the schools are impossibly high. Today a school is expected not only to teach, but also to oversee morality, discipline, discrimination, sex education, health, psychiatric counselling, career placement, and even babysitting. Parents have demanding careers and little time for children. The school is the parents' and society's solution; but the task is too big. This job is to be done for more and more children, with less and less funds, and fewer and fewer accepted rules. It is a losing battle which is becoming acknowledged as such.

We talked with the truant officer about a natural solution—that of parents becoming much more involved with their children. As careers become more boring, one's self becomes more fascinating; as one's self becomes more boring, one's family becomes more fascinating. As one's family becomes more fascinating, parents gladly acknowledge their responsibility for all aspects of their children's learning. Then family and school rejoice. This, we explained, was our experience and our intent. The officer left thanking us for taking such good care of our children. She said the school couldn't do better than we were doing for Eliza.

The home contributes to society directly and indirectly. Its influence helps society's attitudes to become unintentionally accepting; society's words grow coincidentally generous and understanding; its purpose, increasingly balancing. As this change becomes obvious to schools and other social organizations, mutual respect replaces suspicion, apathy, and conflict.

Society is looking for the solutions to its paradoxical problems—the family exploring natural education presents such a solution. The family's attitudes toward its children and the school offers a very real and viable answer at a time when society is becoming particularly open to such a response.

For our family, the evolution of natural education is a process which has barely begun. What it is now is very different from what it must become, but there is no way back to formal education. Our adventure is before us.

For many children, formal education stands in the way of learning. It can distract them from their real teachers. For there is no lack of real teachers in this life, and no scarcity of curiosity, fascination, and flexibility in children. Put the two together—that's all you need. A child becomes like a plant which turns toward the sun. It grows orderly, beautifully, and radiantly for all to enjoy.

Michio Kushi's New School

BY PAULA RUBIRA

"We propose a school that teaches the unification of all antagonistic opposites; those who pass through this school will be noticeable for their health, their ability to create order, and their high judgment. They will be the ones to fully realize a world event of great magnitude which is only beginning in our lifetimes—the meeting of East and West."

T *he following essay rewords and summarizes some of Michio Kushi's ideas on education. It is based primarily on notes taken by Ann LaFlair at a seminar given by Mr. Kushi in July, 1971, in which he outlined a plan for the education of children. Portions of the essay are drawn from Mr. Kushi's writings, and from notes taken at other seminars.*

Let us consider a possible program for the education of our children which is divided into twelve levels, the students' ages corresponding at each level to the current system of education in the United States—that is, beginning at around age six and ending at around age eighteen. There are five basic areas of study: 1) Nature (physics, chemistry, biology); 2) Humanity and society; 3) Creative skills (language, literature, art, music, and technology); 4) Mathematics; 5) Daily life (physical education and home economics).

In the first grade, children learn about the complementary opposites yin and yang as revealed in basic phenomena of nature: shapes, colors, tastes, movement. Instruction in the area of humanity and society is presented in combination with literature, by reading the children stories and fairy tales that also serve to develop the imagination. A sense of fellowship with all cultures is encouraged by singing songs from all over the world. Meditation is practiced at the start of each day in every grade. The alphabet and numbers are repeatedly chanted aloud in unison, for chanting improves circulation and develops physical keenness. The essential rudiments of social behavior—how to greet parents and elders, how to express gratitude and to apologize—are taught along with such practical skills as personal hygiene and keeping the school environment clean and orderly. It is important that children learn to create order from the beginning of their school experience. In each grade level, most classroom work is done in the morning, leaving the afternoons free for agricultural outings, sports events, etc. There should be ample time for outdoor play, as well as origami, painting, writing, drawing, and other creative activities. Students at this level begin to learn the use of various art media—pencils, crayons, watercolors, oils, and black and white brush work—in a progressive order of difficulty, with the medium changing every second year. And, at mealtime, they learn to chew their food well and to eat peacefully.

Children in the second grade study yin and yang in nature—directions, weight, temperature, polarity (plus and minus), etc.; and in daily life—cold versus hot baths, sweet versus salty toothpaste, eating from yang to yin at mealtimes. Teachers continue reading aloud to them, emphasizing fairy tales and imaginative literature.

In the third grade, students learn about yin and yang in the environment (for example, seasonal changes), in the human body (such as in organs and bones), in their social surroundings (relationships among peers, elders, parents, siblings, students and teachers), and in creative skills, especially language and literature. Students are taught to read aloud—a practice to be continued in the higher grades, since this aids the development of clear speech and provides the same physical benefits as unison chanting. Again teachers read aloud to the students, but the selections are now chosen from the best writing of all cultures (the Bible and Confucious, for instance). The children grow their own vegetable garden and begin to make tools and instruments.

In the fourth grade, children study yin and yang in animals, plants, the cycles of the moon and winds, in the development of life forms, basic classification, and in many other aspects of their environment. They begin a study of foreign languages which will continue throughout their school years. They learn to play the flute (the simplest instrument—the greatest art), and study interior decorating and domestic skills like washing clothes and dishes.

Fifth graders study material yin and yang, the physics of temperature and pressure, and states of change. Scale measurements and geometry are added to their mathematical studies. Their social studies extend to the community. Composition, grammar, and poetry are stressed. There is an emphasis on team sports and martial arts, as well as basic cooking—the preparation of bread, rice, and vegetables.

In the sixth grade, nature studies focus upon biological life. The social view expands to encompass the country as a whole, examining the interrelationships of transportation, economic, and political systems.

From the seventh grade, at puberty, boys and girls begin to diverge in their studies, except in certain basic areas. However, the option is always open for them to study subjects in which they have a strong interest, for instance, girls can learn carpentry and boys, sewing. In the seventh grade students learn about the non-material world, or energy—the spirit. They study yin and yang as reflected in the dialectics of world history, in literature, and in composition. They begin making furniture, and learn other manual skills; the garden they planted as third-graders now includes grains as well as vegetables.

Students in the eighth grade are encouraged to express themselves creatively in sculpture, painting, poetry, and music. Working with black and white brush painting—the simplest, most difficult art medium—they are taught to strive towards the ultimate goal of art: to express the largest in the smallest, infinity in the infinitesimal, the highest art evoking infinite nothingness.

Ninth graders study yin and yang in the solar system, the galaxies, the universe; in the rise and fall of ancient civilizations; in such mechanical technologies as motors and power sources; and in domestic economics—saving, budgets, income management.

In the tenth grade, perhaps the most conceptual year of their education, students learn the laws of change as a whole; how to develop health, social peace, and justice; the motivations and origins of technology and politics. They are encouraged to begin to define their own individual dream, their own philosophy of life.

The last two years merge into a single course, designed as a transition into society. There are many directions a student might follow in these years: exchange programs with foreign students; the publishing of books, articles, poetry; art exhibits; work-study programs; farming; studies in domestic life—birth, child-care, home medicine; meditation and philosophy; community planning; archaeology; wilderness expeditions; crafts of all kinds. Each student is given the opportunity to follow his or her own personal dream.

It should be evident from this outline, which points out only the salient features of the curriculum at each grade level, that we study all those subjects ordinarily taught in modern schools, besides many more. There are no tests and no grades. Individual students are evaluated according to the following criteria: Are they healthy? Are they creative? Are they orderly? Do they relate well to others? Do they have behavior problems?

Freedom requires self-discipline. Our aim is to develop this quality in each student. The way for the teacher to handle disruptive behavior is to apologize in front of the class for the misbehaving classmate. The teacher must assume responsibility for everything that happens in his or her classroom. This approach causes the disruptive student to feel remorseful and reestablishes a sense of unity in the class.

The teacher's responsibility also extends to mealtimes. A cafeteria-style arrangement is most suitable. It is the teacher's task to determine the special dietary needs of each pupil: some may need eggs or fish; some may need more or less salt. Meals for children should be cooked with a minimum of salt, and salted condiments made available in the form of gomasio, tamari, etc. The teacher always eats with his or her students, sitting with different children each day so that he or she may observe their eating patterns and make recommendations.

The process of education is threefold: first, unification of mental, physical, and spiritual growth through proper eating in harmony with the natural order; second, discovery of one's own individual dream by exercising the imagination and recognizing that all of life is play; third, contemplation of the laws of change—the Order of the Universe—through intuition. The passive (yin) aspect of intuition is judgment; the active (yang) aspect is will. The quality of our intuition, judgment, and will, and the spirit with which we approach life, depend ultimately upon the quality of the food we eat. When a person has developed sound intuition, a high level of judgment, and a strong will, that person is free.

The school should provide an atmosphere of fun and play. Teachers must be imaginative in their search for ways to present all subjects in this spirit. For example, sports can be used not only as physical education, but also as lessons in mathematics, measuring distance and time. Nature trips can be used for countless studies besides biology. Learning should be an adventure which students will desire to continue long after their formal schooling has ended.

The Large View

Youth and Age: A Broken Exchange

BY STEVIE DANIELS

Most of us can remember older people who gave crucial guidance to younger people by warning them before or helping them after an impulsive blunder in the stormy, confusing years of youth. We can also recall hearing encouraging stories from grandmothers and grandfathers about ancestors who led adventurous and independent lives. Even if we missed such valuable lessons from elders in our own family, we found them in literature and art—for instance, the speech by Grandfather in William Faulkner's *The Reivers*, the remarks of the old Indian chief in *Little Big Man*, exchanges between various characters in *Roots*, or even the homilies of Mammy in *Gone With The Wind*. With these scenes in mind, it is a jolt to realize that 1,200,000 of those over sixty-five in the United States today are consigned to nursing homes, where they are virtually isolated from the young.

Why? When did this separation between young and old begin, and how has it spread?

The increasing relegation of elders to "homes for the aged" since 1940 is the most obvious sign of the widening gap between youth and age. No statistics are available on where older people lived before that time, but within my own memory (and that of many others my age and older) they normally were provided for through the resources of the extended family, especially in the South and other parts of the country which remained centered on farming. Also, certain ethnic groups (especially Blacks, Italians, and Jews) clustered together in large families that tended to retain old customs. The young cared for the old in their homes, and rarely was an older family member sent off to a boarding house or institution.

Causes contributing to the decrease in traditional respect for older family members began to appear at the same time as did revolutionary changes in the American diet and technological advances which transformed our agricultural society into an industrial one. Although mandatory retirement ages, greater social mobility, and the emphasis on higher education also have had their effect, the changes in what we eat and how it is grown have been the main factors in splitting apart the generations.

The dietary change was towards a much higher consumption of meat, dairy products, sugar, refined flour, canned or frozen products, and convenience foods. The new dietary pattern was accompanied by the invention and marketing of many gadgets for the modern kitchen, designed to get a meal on the table "in a wink." This trend dramatically reduced the amount of care and physical contact that the person preparing a family's meals put into cooking. As the meal was prepared in a hurry, it was also consumed in a rush, and the ageless tradition of the whole family eating a leisurely meal together began to disappear. With that linchpin gone, the axle uniting all the generations of one family began to wobble and go askew. Often members didn't eat the same food, each one grabbing a bite in a different snackbar or lunchroom. As our diets moved away from whole, natural foods prepared in the family kitchen toward processed foods and meals served in restaurants the decomposition of the family unit accelerated, and the phrase "generation gap" began to appear frequently in the media.

Until the turn of the century, America was predominantly agricultural, with cohesive family units that lived in close proximity, engaged in common efforts, and shared similar interests. The older members of these units were regarded as sources of wisdom and practical knowledge (specifically in the essential crafts such as making clothes and furniture, building houses, etc.). Even when these elders could no longer contribute much physical energy they were still crucial to the group's survival. The younger members became responsible for the land, under the guidance of the elders, who shared the home until their death.

With the changeover to industrialism, many young family members moved into the cities, and few returned to the farm. Without enough hands to work the land, small farms began to disappear under the onslaught of agribusiness. Eventually, there was no homestead to which the young could return, even if they had wanted to. The resulting geographical gap between young and old accelerated the trend toward members of the same family living in separate locations scattered throughout the states.

For many immigrant groups, the separation between elders living in the country and younger people living in the city took the form of elders being left behind in the "old country" while the younger generation lived quite different lives in the "new world." Among the ethnic family groups in American cities, the gap between generations gradually widened as the children learned skills more and more in public school and less and less from elders. They began to view their parents, who often spoke little or no English, as ignorant and out of place in the society to which they were adapting.

The lack of a common spiritual network in the United States also contributed to the breakdown in communication between old and young. With no traditional rituals to define specific interactions between them, the generations became puzzled about their relationship to each other. In older, more conservative cultures such as India, Japan, and China, the patterns have been ritualized for centuries and, even though the family unit is starting to deteriorate in those parts of the world also, strong family bonds are still functional there.

In America, of course, there are still many members of the younger generation willing and able to care for and learn from their parents. Unfortunately, that natural custom is being eroded by the factors we have mentioned earlier—revolutionary changes in dietary, farming, and cultural patterns—all leading toward increasing abandonment of the older population to nursing homes or similar institutions. The young are faced with the difficult task of caring for elders, many of whom have lost their physical health and feel useless because their advice has become irrelevant in a rapidly changing world. As the younger generation begins to suffer increasingly from the chronic diseases caused by modern dietary patterns and unhealthy lifestyles, many of them have become physically and emotionally unable to care for elderly relatives and therefore turn to nursing homes as a symptomatic solution for their dilemma.

However, institutionalization is clearly not a viable solution. In addition to the disastrous cultural effects of separating a society from its elders, the elders are not even adequately cared for in these institutions. Countless independent and government studies have shown that most nursing homes have poor fire protection, unsatisfactory sanitary conditions, insufficient staffing, poorly prepared and nutritionally inadequate food, and no protection for residents from the thievery of others.

We have been undergoing a transition period from extended families, centered in rural settings, to nuclear families (and other social forms) separated from other families by highly specialized occupations and widely disparate incomes. There are, however, some tentative signs that the pendulum may be swinging back. The growing interest in natural foods, the search for appropriate uses of technology, the increase in handmade items, and the efforts by small groups to replenish the soil through natural and organic farming all give evidence of a turn in the cycle.

Hopefully, studying those aspects of our daily lives that connect us to our ancestors will give us a broader view of the importance and need for younger members to assist and learn from their elders. Even in traditional cultures where the family was not the primary social unit, the elders were honored. Many Indo-European, American Indian,

African, and South American tribal groups centered their social organization around a body of older members.

By strengthening ourselves through healthier lifestyles and diets (in a family or other community grouping) we will begin to restore those traditions which make our lives whole, such as bearing our children at home, preparing and eating our food together at home, and dying at home as part of the natural process of life.

We can also bring aging back to the home.

By returning to a diet of whole, natural foods we will begin to restore the continuity with each other, our ancestors, and the earth. By building extended families, either through the community around us or by having children and inviting our parents to join us, we can bridge the generation gap. We can take the first step toward regaining physical, emotional, and spiritual health for ourselves and the future.

Be Fruitful and Multiply

BY BRUCE DONEHOWER

In contrast to the mostly subdued houses in suburban Lexington, Massachusetts, the Soparkar home is brightly lit and radiates vitality on this cold winter evening in February. The house seems to be throwing off sparks of activity as we walk up the path to the front door.

We are met by two of the daughters, who show us inside where a group of curious young faces, ranging in age from three to twenty-one, smile at us and wonder what we've come to talk to them about. A fire is started in the living room fireplace while we wait for the father, Bob Soparkar, to return from his weekly trip to the open-air vegetable market in Boston. Their curiosities satisfied, some of the younger children are sent off to bed, supervised by their older siblings.

Years ago a large family would have attracted no attention, while today we question the judgment of anyone who chooses to have more than two kids. The Soparkars have fourteen, four of their own and the rest adopted from Central and South America. A family this large must certainly raise some eyebrows.

Bob Soparkar, an orthodontist and dental researcher, admits that his professional friends have trouble understanding his motives.

"When people find out we have fourteen children they usually ask how we manage, meaning: 'We know damn well you can't manage with so many children so what are you doing?' I always answer that it depends what your thinking is. My wife and I don't think we are doing anyone any favors. Nobody is forcing us to have a large family, we do it because we enjoy it."

As he talks the children who are present listen attentively but do not interrupt. No one is restless.

The father goes on to explain that he was born in India where a large, extended family is a way of life. His uncles all had six or seven children. When he visited them he was welcomed into their families as though he were their own child. He could stay with them as long as he wanted, and no one thought anything of it.

"Growing up in a large family, with many people around, teaches youngsters to respect each other's rights and to honor them," Soparkar explains. "When kids leave a large family, they are better able to get along with other people because they understand the value of compromise and give and take. In smaller families these lessons are only words. Kids need to learn from experience."

"You learn social skills in a family this size," adds the Soparkar's oldest daughter. "Skills like patience, how to get along with other people, how to listen and express yourself."

"And how to laugh," says the mother.

Mrs. Beryl Soparkar, a native New Englander, smiles when we ask about her family background. She explains that she was an only child who always felt lonely. Having many people around her to share with was a dream she had had from an early age.

"A family this size teaches skills in all tasks to all children," she adds. "We think it also promotes self-sufficiency and broadens one's views and one's appreciation of others. Our multicultural experiences and backgrounds help to keep our minds open and receptive, too."

As she speaks a minor ruckus breaks out in the kitchen. No one is too concerned. The feeling seems to be that everyone is watching out for each other. The older children care for the younger. Despite the many different energies in the household, the overall feeling is one of calm and well-being.

"There is more openness in a large family," says Mrs. Soparkar. "Having so many different personalities around means that you are free to be yourself."

When asked about the children's educational expenses, the Soparkars admit that this is a problem. Yet, they point out, with inflation running the way it is, sending even one child to college is difficult for any family. They talk about the alternatives to higher education and the chances of scholarships or working one's way through school, which their oldest daughter is presently doing. No one seems too anxious about the future.

"It takes a lot of very sensitive attunement to each child to help maintain individuality and to provide just that very set of lessons or experiences which will mean the most to that child," Mrs. Soparkar tells us.

"Each of us does our own thing, and yet we all help each other and feel pride in each other," adds the oldest son.

"What about medical expenses?"

"We don't get sick," replies Mrs. Soparkar simply. "In this family sickness is not reinforced. No one has time to dote on you if you are sick. Also, we've been involved with natural foods for a long time, at least twenty years, way back before I was pregnant with the first child. We avoid junk food, and there is no sugar in the house.''

In the kitchen, she shows us a broken freezer which she has stocked with grains and beans. The boxes of fresh vegetables from the open air market are piled one on top of another, waiting to be sorted .

''Are you planning to adopt any more children?'' we ask her as we depart.

''Not for the time being,'' she answers, smiling.

We get the feeling that she wouldn't mind if they did.

Do You Know Who Your Great-Grandparents Were?
A Discussion of Family Roots

BY MICHIO KUSHI

Families are of two kinds: horizontal and vertical. Horizontal families center on the relationship between husband and wife; vertical families stress the continuity between ancestors and descendants. Whereas the vertical is the traditional form, the horizontal is a modern phenomenon.

A more horizontal structure is typical of the United States. In this structure, the husband and wife form a more or less independent unit. Of course, there may be friendly, social relations between the families of brothers and sisters, but they are not very deep.

This horizontal pattern is typical of modern industrialized nations, where the preoccupation in life tends to be the individual's way of earning a living. That emphasis dates from about the seventeenth century. People in the modern world go where there is work, and the resulting mobility acts as a disintegrating factor on the ties between brothers, sisters, and other relatives. As those links weaken, the traditions uniting family members gradually disappear; very few people today know much about their great-grandparents or even grandparents. Thus the lifespan of any one horizontal family is very short, normally encompassing only two or, at most, three generations.

Extending over countless generations, the unity of the vertical family is maintained by three factors: dietary, spiritual, and practical. This vertical form is still the general rule in the Orient—in China, India, Indonesia, Japan, and Southeast Asia.

Dietary unity means that the family has a typical style of cooking. Since we are what we eat, all the generations in such families tend to resemble each other in physique and personality. Their characteristic way of eating is maintained by the custom of a bride's coming to live with the groom's parents for two or three months before the wedding in order to learn the family's typical cooking methods. After she has learned how to carry on the family's traditional diet, the new couple is free to set up a household on its own.

This physiological unity is reinforced by a spiritual practice emphasizing reverence for ancestors. A quiet room is normally set aside in the main home of the extended family, where some type of shrine, no matter how simple, is dedicated to the spirits of deceased family members. The head of the house meditates or prays there every morning and evening. Each branch of the family has a miniature of this shrine in its house, and members of the branch family pay their respects to it daily. Even if some of the branch families live far away, the whole clan gathers every year or so for a reunion. These celebrations normally include some kind of memorial ceremony or acknowledgment of the ancestors.

The biological and spiritual unity is further cemented by a set of shared norms, which particularly apply when choosing marriage partners. These norms include agreed-upon standards of behavior, such as honesty, ethical business practices, the enjoyment of simple pleasures, etc. The Mosaic code, which unified all the Jewish tribes, is an example of that custom within the Western tradition.

In the vertical family, parents and often grandparents initiate children into the family's ethical heritage by praising or pointing out the inadequacy of the children's behavior in terms of that code and its precedents. If one member of a vertical family gets into trouble, the older members assemble for a family council. If a particular individual, for example, is put in jail for some offense, they decide whether to work for his release and how to go about it, or whether to let him remain in jail as a justified lesson. On the contrary, if one member receives an unusual honor, the whole family feels proud and throws a big party to celebrate.

In the vertical family, a spouse is selected with everyone's participation and approval, because the new couple will be carrying on the traditions of a much larger unit than itself. In forming a horizontal family, the young couple may ask for their parents' opinions, but in most cases the real decision has already been made. To a certain extent, members of a horizontal family may share some spiritual unity through their religion, but that also tends to be a minor factor. As for dietary unity, it has been almost completely lost through the massive modern changeover to commercially prepared food.

Both the horizontal and the vertical patterns have their advantages and disadvantages. However, I feel that too much stress in recent times has been placed on the advantages of the horizontal family and the disadvantages of the vertical family. It is worth keeping in mind that, although maintaining a vertical structure involves certain difficulties, those very obstacles can be taken as challenges inherent in extending the game of life to include many generations rather than two or three generations isolated in geographical space.

For anyone who is interested in restoring the unity of his or her vertical family, I would like to suggest beginning with the following practice: Start to write a history of your family. Where did your parents, grandparents, and ancestors come from? What kinds of things did they do? What kind of people were they? Try to find out their places of birth and death and all their children's names. Then give copies of this record to your own children, advising them to extend it further. That way you can rekindle an interest in the traditional family and pass it on to future generations.

A Bibliography

BY BARBARA JACOBS

T he following book list is not a definitive one on the subjects of pregnancy, childbirth, and child care. Rather, it is a brief introduction to some of the books I've found most useful during my five pregnancies. Of course, no matter how helpful a book might be, it can never substitute for human advice and real experience. In addition, each pregnancy and birth is unique, and so there are no absolutes. Common sense and flexibility are the most important guidelines.

The Macrobiotic Guidebook for Living *by Georges Ohsawa (Los Angeles: Ohsawa Foundation, 1965), 128 pages, paperback, $1.50.*

Ohsawa's unique approach makes the *Guidebook for Living* a very worthwhile book concerning all aspects of family life. It is the original macrobiotic manual of love, marriage, pregnancy, and child-raising, and while it is written from a Japanese point of view and may not be totally applicable to Americans, the **Guidebook** is very inspiring and contains a good deal of practical information.

From Conception to Birth *by Roberts Rugh and Landrum B. Shettles, M.D. (New York: Harper & Row, 1971), 262 pages, hardcover, $15.00.*

I thought I'd glance through this book casually, but I was immediately caught up in the fascinating and readable day-by-day account of embryological and fetal development, accompanied by drawings and color photographs. This first section was written by Rugh, an embryologist; the second section, written by his colleague, an obstetrician, is far less interesting. Shettles seems to be one of those doctors who insist on making all the decisions. Fortunately this attitude is becoming somewhat dated, as many of us are beginning to rely more on ourselves, alternative healers, and friends than on so-called experts. He does provide some useful information and facts, but because of his authoritarian position I would much rather get that information from some other source. I do recommend this book, however, for its first section and especially for the fine photographs and illustrations.

Life before Birth *by Ashley Montague (New York: New American Library, 1964), 256 pages, paperback, $1.25.*

Many statistics and much medical data provide the reader with a vast assortment of information on the relationship of the mother's age, diet, activity, general health, and emotional condition to her child's development before birth.

Macrobiotic Pregnancy *by Alice Feinberg (Los Angeles: Georges Ohsawa Macrobiotic Foundation, 1973), 78 pages, paperback, $1.50.*

This short book covers a wide range of topics related to pregnancy and baby care. It will be a valuable aid for anyone interested in using natural techniques in accordance with macrobiotic philosophy.

Macrobiotic Childcare *by Cornellia Aihara (Chico, Calif.: Georges Ohsawa Macrobiotic Foundation, 1971), 42 pages, paperback, $1.50.*

Mrs. Aihara presents a very warm account of her own experience raising children according to macrobiotic philosophy.

Husband-coached Childbirth *by Robert A. Bradley, M.D. (New York: Harper & Row, 1965), 214 pages, hardcover, $7.95.*

This is the basic book for those women whose husbands have yet to get involved in the birth experience. Although it's now dated, it does have its place as a source book for those couples planning to have their children in the hospital.

The Experience of Childbirth *by Sheila Kitzinger (Middlesex, England: Penguin Books, 1972), 280 pages, paperback, $1.95.*

This is my favorite among childbirth books. Written in a very personal and encouraging manner, it includes an excellent section on "Learning Harmony in Labor" for relaxing during labor. Ms. Kitzinger has five children herself, so the book is certainly coming from extensive personal experience.

9 months, 1 year, 1 day *written by parents, compiled by Jean Marzollo (New York: Harper & Row, 1975), 191 pages, hardcover, $7.95.*

A practical, informative, and entertaining collection of ideas on all aspects of pregnancy and baby care, this compilation is good light reading for a pregnant woman.

Essential Exercises for the Childbearing Years *by Elizabeth Noble, R.P.T. (Boston: Houghton Mifflin, 1976), 180 pages, $4.95.*

Developed by a physical therapist, these exercises are based on the progression of physical changes which take place during the childbearing period.

Midwifery by Jean L. Hallum (New York: Arco Publishing Co., 1972), 152 pages, paperback, $5.00.

Originally a text for obstetric nurses and midwives, this concise book deals with pregnancy from a medical point of view. Although it discusses complications of pregnancy and labor, it keeps in mind that childbirth is a natural occurrence which normally necessitates little or no outside intervention. A few of the topics discussed are female anatomy, fertilization and fetal development, blood types, and the physiology of pregnancy.

Spiritual Midwifery by Ina May and The Farm Midwives (Summertown, Tenn.: The Book Publishing Co., 1975), 380 pages, paperback, $5.95.

The women of the Farm, a Tennessee commune, convey the joy of childbirth in telling their personal experiences. The drawings and photographs are beautiful and inspiring. In addition to descriptions of the births both by mothers and by their attending midwives, the book contains sections on care of the newborn and instructions for midwives.

Immaculate Deception by Suzanne Arms (Boston: San Francisco Book Co./Houghton Mifflin, 1975), 318 pages, hardcover, $11.95.

Immaculate Deception, a harsh, detailed exposé of hospital childbirth and maternity care practices in America, is a very powerful, unsentimental book. If you are considering a homebirth, this book will reinforce your most positive views about it; if you are considering a hospital birth, it will stimulate many questions.

Birth Without Violence by Frederick Leboyer (New York: Alfred A. Knopf, 1975), 174 pages, hardcover, $8.95.

The remarkably beautiful photographs of newborn infants that accompany Leboyer's text strongly support his argument against the unnecessary pain and trauma that are often part of the birth experience. Already something of a classic, this book should be read by every pregnant woman. Leboyer's startlingly simple techniques actually work; you owe it to your child.

Loving Hands by Frederick Leboyer (New York: Alfred A. Knopf, 1976), 139 pages, hardcover, $7.95.

This book elaborates on the massage technique briefly mentioned in *Birth Without Violence*. Photographs illustrate the poetic instructions for massage of the new baby according to traditional Asian Indian methods.

Nursing Your Baby *by Karen Pryor (New York: Harper & Row, 1975), 289 pages, paperback, $1.95.*

Of the many books available on breastfeeding, I've found *Nursing Your Baby* one of the most informative and readable. Even an experienced mother could probably learn something from the information packed in this book on all aspects of nursing, from prenatal care to weaning a toddler. The scientific information provided is never overly technical—the book is like a knowledgeable friend, practical and personal.

Breastfeeding and Natural Child-Spacing *by Sheila Kippley (New York: Penguin Books, 1975), 197 pages, paperback, $2.95.*

This book, devoted entirely to the aspect of breastfeeding that the author calls "natural infertility," is the first of its kind. Natural birth control through nursing is not a new idea, however; traditional cultures have known and utilized this fact for centuries, and today it is an appealing alternative to artificial contraception. Ms. Kippley's topics include the entire range of breastfeeding experience, from nursing a newborn through weaning an older baby.

Biography of the Unborn *by Margaret Shea Gilbert (Hafner Publishing Co., Inc. 1962), 160 pages, hardcover.*

Very readable classic on embryological development.

Pregnancy, Birth and the Newborn Baby *by Boston Children's Medical Center and Richard Feinbloom, M.D. (Delta Publishing Co., Inc., 1971), 471 pages, paperback, $8.95.*

Good standard medical primer.

How to Raise a Healthy Child in Spite of Your Doctor *by Robert Mendelsohn, M.D. (Contemporary Books, 1984), 244 pages, hardcover, $14.95.*

Macrobiotic Pregnancy and Care of the Newborn *by Michio and Aveline Kushi (Japan Publications, 1984), 264 pages, paperback, $14.95.*

Birthing Normally *by Gayle Peterson Mindbody Press (Berkeley, 1984), 253 pages, paperback, $10.95.*

Childbirth Wisdom *by Judith Goldsmith (Congdon & Weed, 1984), 256 pages, paperback, $18.95.*

This wonderful book is filled with the wisdom of traditional cultures from around the world. Drawing on childbirth lore, customs, and practices that have been passed from woman to woman in tribal societies, the author is able to present practical and wonderful practices which will make for a joyous, healthful and happy pregnancy and childbirth.

Birth Reborn *by Dr. Michel Odent, Pantheon (New York, 1984), hardcover, $15.95.*

The Roots of Love *by Helene S. Arnstein (New York: Bobbs-Merrill, 1975), 228 pages, hardcover, $7.95.*
A very enjoyable book that covers the first three years of childhood from a psychological point of view, it's the kind of book you might like to read while nursing your baby and dreaming about his or her future.

The Sufi Message *of Hazrat Inayat Khan, vol. 3 (London: Barrie and Rockliff, 1960), 262 pages, hardcover, $5.50.*
Volume 3 of Khan's work concerns the Sufi philosophy of education, character-building, the art of personality, and moral culture. One of the few books to present child development from a spiritual and poetic point of view, it gave me deep insight into the invisible origins of my children.

An excellent catalog of books on Birth and Parenting can be obtained from Orange Cat, 442 Church Street, Garberville, CA 95440. They list over one hundred books which can be purchased directly from them.

A

amesake, 177 – 178, 83
anemia, 33, 56, 95
anemic, 34 – 36
Apgar test, 120
aspirin, 142

B

bacteria, 134, 139
bancha tea, 63, 169
birth control, 12, 70
breastfeeding, 12, 16,
64, 66, 68, 72, 74, 75,
84, 86, 87, 93, 100, 214
burns, 150

C

Caesarean section, 10
calcium, 6, 8, 12, 27, 29,
79, 119
carob, 167
cause of sickness, 124
chicken pox, 130, 148
childbirth, 10, 27, 66,
73, 210 – 210
childhood illnesses,
129, 147, 132
chirimen iriko, 35
chlorophyll plaster, 153
choosing a doctor, 144
circumcision, 9, 59
cold, 150
cookies, 160, 164, 167,
169, 170, 172, 173, 178,
179
cravings, 119
cuts, 150

D

daikon tea, 144, 151
dessert, 164, 167, 176,
178
diaper rash, 122, 39

diet, 3 – 8, 16, 25, 30,
33, 36 – 38, 41, 58, 63,
64, 68, 72, 76, 80, 94,
97 – 98, 105 – 106,
112 – 114, 119 – 123,
125, 128, 137, 139, 147,
150, 158, 199, 202
diphtheria, 131, 135,
149
doctors, 10, 4, 41, 64,
68, 74, 100, 127 – 130,
137 – 139, 144, 145
dulse, 35

E

ears, 121
endogenous pyrogen,
141

F

feeding, 12
fever, 19, 122, 140

G

germs, 134
ginger compress, 152
gluten, 165 – 166

H

hara maki, 28
hernia, 18
hiziki condiment, 31
homebirth, 6, 55, 74
humors, 142
hypothalamus, 141

I

immunizations, 106,
124, 126, 127, 130, 133,
144
infectious diseases, 124
iron, 28, 31, 33, 35, 141
IUD, 12, 13, 47, 49, 51

J

juice, 167, 175, 178, 179

K

kanten, 167, 178
koi – koku, 37, 63
kokkoh, 81
Kushi, 3, 5, 103, 111,
13, 150, 193, 214
kuzu, 151

L

labor, 11
lactation, 102
Leboyer method, 11
lotus root tea, 151
lunches, 157 – 159, 161,
163
lymph system, 148

M

Macrobiotics, 3, 5, 13,
17, 27, 29, 150, 153
measles, 18, 130, 131,
135, 149
meningitis, 141
midwife, 6, 30, 31, 55,
56, 74, 91, 92, 94
mochi, 36, 63
morning sickness, 29
mumps, 130, 135, 149
mustard plaster, 152

N

natural childbirth, 9
natural immunity, 126,
128, 135
nursing, 3, 9, 37 – 38,
45, 55, 63 – 68, 72 – 75,
77 – 80, 83 – 87, 121,
199, 201, 211 – 213

E*ast West Journal*, one of the nation's principal magazines advocating the importance of a healthful diet, has been published for fourteen years from Brookline, Massachusetts. Long before it became fashionable to dine on granola, yoghurt, and tofu, *East West Journal* was stressing the value of eating less saturated fats and more fiber and complex carbohydrates. The value of eating whole and natural foods is one of the primary topics of every issue of *EWJ*.

In addition, *East West Journal* has focused primarily on the quality of life and simple ways to maintain health. Each issue of the magazine has presented practical methods of preventing sickness, from childhood to old age, and natural ways to relieve the symptoms of disease. The magazine has regularly featured articles on childcare, many of which are included in this book.

East West Journal is a magazine with an objective: The holistic quality of life...physical, spiritual, and intellectual.

The writers of the *Journal* are people you can trust and rely on. They are people who have made a natural lifestyle their own. And they write on everything from organic gardening, wilderness trekking, and long distance running, to spinning yarn, making your own pickles, and raising children naturally.

EWJ is available in selected natural foods stores and bookstores throughout the U.S. and Europe. Subscriptions are available for only $18.00 for one year. Please address your subscription order to *East West Journal* P.O. Box 1200, Department W, 17 Station Street, Brookline, Massachusetts 02147.

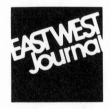